Quality indicators for general prac

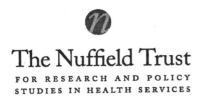

The Nuffield Trust

FOR RESEARCH AND POLICY
STUDIES IN HEALTH SERVICES

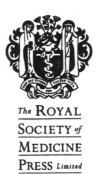

The ROYAL
SOCIETY of
MEDICINE
PRESS Limited

Quality indicators for general practice

A practical guide to clinical quality indicators for primary care health professionals and managers

Edited by

Martin Marshall

General Practitioner and Professor of General Practice

Stephen Campbell

Research Fellow

Jenny Hacker

Research Technician

Martin Roland

General Practitioner and Professor of General Practice

National Primary Care Research and Development Centre
University of Manchester

1 Wimpole Street, London W1G 0AE, UK
207 Westminster Road, Lake Forest, IL, 60045, USA
www.rsmpress.co.uk

British Libaray Catologuing in Publication Data
A catalogue record for this book is available from the British Library

ISBN: 1-85315-488-1

Typeset by Phoenix Photosetting, Chatham, Kent
                                                lasgow
Printed and bound in Great Britain by
Marston Lindsay Ross International Ltd,
Oxfordshire

▶ Contents

▶ List of contributors

Stephen Campbell
Research Fellow, National Primary Care Research and Development Centre, University of Manchester

Jean Coope
General Practitioner, Bollington, Cheshire

Brendan Delaney
Senior Lecturer, Department of Primary Care and General Practice, University of Birmingham

Tom Fahey
Senior Lecturer, Department of Primary Care, University of Bristol

Adrian Freeman
Research Fellow, Institute of General Practice, University of Exeter

Jenny Hacker
Research Technician, National Primary Care Research and Development Centre, University of Manchester

Michael Hall
Honorary Fellow, University of Exeter and Chair, Diabetes UK

Nicholas Hicks
Director of Public Health, Oxfordshire Health Authority

Pali Hungin
Professor, Centre for Health Studies, University of Durham

Tony Kendrick
Professor of Primary Medical Care, University of Southampton

Tim Lancaster
Lecturer in General Practice, Department of Primary Health Care, University of Oxford

Paul Little
MRC Clinician Scientist and Senior Lecturer, Primary Medical Care Group, University of Southampton

David Mant
Professor of General Practice, Department of Primary Health Care, University of Oxford

Martin Marshall
Professor of General Practice, National Primary Care Research and Development Centre, University of Manchester

Stephen Morgan
Senior Clinical Research Fellow, Department of Primary Medical Care, University of Southampton

Norma O'Flynn
NHS R&D National Primary Care Training Fellow, Division of Primary Care and Public Health Sciences, Guy's, King's and St Thomas' School of Medicine

Sarah Purdy
Lecturer, Department of Primary Health Care, University of Newcastle upon-Tyne

Leone Ridsdale
Reader, Division of Primary Care and Public Health Sciences, Guy's, King's and St Thomas' School of Medicine

Martin Roland
Professor of General Practice and Director, National Primary Care Research and Development Centre, University of Manchester

Alison Round
Consultant in Public Health Medicine, North and East Devon Health Authority

Clare Seamark
Research Fellow, Institute of General Practice, University of Exeter

Helen Smith
Senior Lecturer, Department of Primary Medical Care, University of Southampton

Martin Underwood
Senior Lecturer, Department of General Practice and Primary Care, Queen Mary College, University of London

Sue Wilson
Senior Lecturer, Department of Primary Care and General Practice, University of Birmingham

▶ How to use this book

This is not a book that you need to read from cover to cover. It is designed as a reference book and practical guide for anyone who works in general practice or is involved in managing the quality of general practice-based clinical care. In Chapter 1 we provide a brief introduction to the concept of quality in general practice. We suggest a working definition of quality, define the term 'quality indicator' and describe the benefits and problems of using quality indicators. In Chapter 2 we describe the development of the quality indicator set. Some of the details are technical in nature but the information will be useful to those who wish to understand the origin of the quality indicators. Chapters 3–21 represent each of the clinical areas for which we developed indicators. Each chapter has been written by a primary care expert in the field and has a similar structure: an outline of why the subject is important; a review of the evidence relating to the final set of indicators; and a full list of references together with some suggested further reading. These chapters provide up-to-date clinical evidence and we hope that many readers will find them a useful educational resource and a teaching aid for those in training for general practice. In Chapter 22 we describe how the indicators may be used for quality assessment and to encourage quality improvement, and also how they should not be used.

▶ Foreword

This guide to clinical quality indicators in general practice is designed as a reference book for anyone who works in general practice or is involved in managing the quality of general practice-based clinical care. The book forms one part of a wider programme of work supported by the Nuffield Trust that focuses on the quality of health care. Quality has been an explicit concern to the Trust for over a decade. In 1990, Gordon McLachlan, former Secretary of the Trust, took as the theme of his Rock Carling Fellowship, *What Price Quality?*[i] In 1998, the Trust co-funded and organised a national conference on quality and organisational change at which the results of a review of quality initiatives in the United Kingdom were presented.[ii] Following this review, the Trust's programme on quality was broadened to take an international perspective to ensure that policy thinking on matters that relate to quality should be informed by the experience of other countries. To achieve this goal, the Trust entered into partnerships with organisations such as the Commonwealth Fund of New York, OECD, WHO and, in particular, with RAND Health. RAND has the largest non-government health care research organisation in the United States and has helped shape responses to emerging healthcare issues over the last three decades. RAND Health's work has focused on the development of rigorous methods to measure and report on quality, the organisation and financing of health systems, and access to care. This research has clearly demonstrated that quality of care can be measured; that quality of care varies enormously as a function of the physician, the healthcare team, and the setting in which the patient is treated; and that deficiencies in quality of care, where they occur, are too great to be ignored.

The Nuffield Trust's collaboration with RAND Health was the subject of a two-day workshop at the Trust in March 1999. At this workshop, a programme of work was developed with the general object of exploring the relevance to the United Kingdom of concepts and empirical investigation developed in the United States. As a result of that meeting, a decision was made to focus on three areas. These areas were the U.S. experience with the public release of comparative information about quality and its relevance to the United Kingdom[iii]; the development and reporting of data on coronary artery bypass surgery; and the subject of this book, the development of quality indicators relevant to British primary care.

The potential benefits of international collaboration are increasingly recognised[iv]. A growing number of countries worldwide perceive a common need to build systemic capacity for safeguarding and improving the quality of health care. While acknowledging the considerable variation in context between countries, it is imperative to explore the role of and potential for cross-national collaboration to advance a common goal of improved performance in health care quality. Often, the conventional basis for collaboration is the perception of similar needs, but we must also identify differences. In this way, we can build on the variations of experience and expertise as well as the commonalities. Divergent legacies and orientations may point to the richest areas for learning through cross-fertilisation to facilitate transfer of insights and expertise.

Building systemic national capacity to remedy and improve quality in health care requires coordination and integration of activity at four levels: national policy formulation, national and system level infrastructure for monitoring and oversight, system level governance and operational management, and clinical provision of services. The United States and the United Kingdom exhibit strengths at different levels. The United Kingdom has national policy and new infrastructure, including the National Institute for Clinical Excellence and the Commission for Health Improvement, and has designed functions for systems level management and monitoring such as the National Service Frameworks and the National Performance Framework. The United States is a leader in quality measurement and reporting largely due to its market approach to health care and consumer orientation designed to provide choice.

This book describes a part of the Nuffield's international collaboration that breaks new ground. In the United Kingdom, particularly in primary care practice, quality assessment is a relatively new area of study, and the introduction of clinical governance and the National Performance Framework suggested that further work to help guide policy and practice should be a priority. The development of primary care quality indicators in the United Kingdom has been led by the National Primary Care Research and Development Centre. This development process is expensive and time-consuming. Thus, it was agreed that it would be worthwhile to explore the possibility that the United Kingdom could achieve a significant advance by transferring measurement technologies from RAND's work in the United States. The project aimed to examine the practical feasibility and policy implications of such an initiative.

Three compelling arguments favor organised international collaboration.[4] First the field of quality evaluation and improvement has universally applicable goals, methods, and intended outputs. Secondly, because the necessary research and development are resource intensive, technology transfer and sharing of expertise are desirable. Thirdly, fair and valid international comparisons are possible only through formal international cooperation. This project and these sets of working documents demonstrate the value of support for international collaboration through systematic assessment and sharing of the experience and expertise of the various countries. This recognition in turn reinforces the need to develop shared languages of measurement and evaluation; implement complementary programmes in each nation, in keeping with its national character and its healthcare culture; and make a long-term commitment to maintaining programmes for mutual benefit. We believe this book will make a significant contribution toward these efforts.

John Wyn Owen CB
Secretary
Nuffield Trust
July 2001

i   McLachlan G. *What Price Quality?*. Nuffield Trust. 1990.
ii Leatherman S, Sutherland K. *Evolving Quality in the new NHS: policy, process and pragmatic considerations*. Nuffield Trust. 1998.

iii   Marshall M, Shekelle P, Brook R, Leatherman S. *Dying to Know: public release of information about quality of health care*. Nuffield Trust 2000.

iv   Leatherman S, Donaldson LJ, Eisenberg JM. "International Collaboration: harnessing differences to meet common needs in improving quality of care". *Quality in Health Care*, 200;9:143-145.

▶ Acknowledgements

We wish to thank the Trustees, Secretary and members of the Quality Steering Group of the Nuffield Trust for the financial support and practical guidance of the project on which this book is based. The project was conducted in collaboration with researchers from the RAND Health Program, Santa Monica, California, in particular Paul Shekelle, Elizabeth McGlynn and Robert Brook. Together, they are responsible for much of the developmental work that gave rise to our quality indicator set. We have learnt much from them and value their contribution and guidance. We are also grateful to other members of the RAND team, too many to mention by name, who contributed to the original US literature reviews and the development of the US indicators from which many of the UK indicators are derived. We thank Sarah Heyes for her administrative support, Sue Kirk and Sandra Kennell-Webb for the preliminary field testing of this set of indicators. Last, but certainly not least, we thank the clinical chapter authors for their hard work and for putting up with our constant editorial demands.

MM
SC
JH
MR

July 2001

►1

Introduction to quality assessment in general practice

Martin Marshall and Stephen Campbell

Key points

► Quality has several different dimensions. Patients, professionals and managers will place different values on these dimensions.

► Improving quality of care is at the centre of the current reforms of the National Health Service.

► Most of the methods that can be used to improve quality are already in everyday use in many practices. The current focus on quality helps to bring these methods together and to adopt a more critical view of the best balance between the approaches.

► Quality indicators represent one way of using information to examine differences in quality against explicit standards, between organisations and over time.

► There are both benefits and risks to using quality indicators to stimulate improvements in quality.

What is quality?

The 'quality agenda' has a high profile in the British National Health Service, as it does in most other developed countries. Quality is, however, a difficult concept to define when applied to health care and efforts to do so in a single sentence are usually misleading and unhelpful. Health care quality has a number of different dimensions. Identifying these helps to clarify the origin of quality problems, potential solutions to the problems and the differing (and sometimes contradictory) perspectives of the people who work in and use health care. Examples of this approach to quality are shown in Boxes 1.1 and 1.2.

Describing quality in terms of its dimensions is particularly helpful to understanding quality in general practice. Patients or users of general practice need to be able to get to (access) a range of services, which should be provided in a professionally competent and humane way (clinical and interpersonal effectiveness). All individuals and groups within a population should get a fair deal (equity) and

---

Box 1.1   The 'structure, process and outcome' model of quality[1]

Structure   The more visible aspects of a health system, e.g. buildings, equipment, trained staff, appointment systems

Process   What goes on within the structure, e.g. consulting, decision making, prescribing, referring

Outcome   The consequences of providing care, e.g. morbidity, mortality, quality of life, user satisfaction and experiences

---

Box 1.2   A multidimensional model of quality[2]

Quality of care for individuals depends on:
  Access
  Clinical effectiveness
  Interpersonal effectiveness

Quality of care for populations depends additionally on:
  Equity
  Efficiency

---

society should get the best value for money taking into account the opportunity costs of resourcing one area at the expense of another (efficiency).

There is, of course, a tension between these different dimensions of quality. Inevitably a trade-off has to be made – it is rarely possible to deliver good quality on all dimensions at the same time. General practitioners might reasonably argue that they could provide better clinical care if resources were put into, say, employing a practice nurse to run a diabetic clinic in their practice. However, this investment might better be made in providing additional community services for mentally ill patients, or reducing waiting lists for an orthopaedic outpatient clinic. In addition there is a very real tension in general practice between the needs (and demands) of individual patients and those of the practice or local community as a whole.

This tension ensures that the debate about quality is often controversial. While we recognise the danger of oversimplifying a complex issue, it is nevertheless helpful to start addressing quality in areas where there is clear evidence of problems[3] and where significant improvements are most likely to be achieved. For this reason this book focuses specifically on the technical processes performed by general practitioners and practice nurses in delivering clinical care for the most common problems presenting to general practice. This pragmatic focus on clinical effectiveness is not meant to divert attention from other important dimensions of quality, particularly interpersonal care – so this book examines only one dimension, albeit an important one, of quality in general practice.

Why is quality important?

So many demands have been made on general practice in the last decade that general practitioners and other members of the primary health care team could be forgiven for dismissing the quality agenda as yet another fad. Some health professionals think that if they ignore current initiatives to improve quality then attention will soon shift elsewhere. This is unlikely to be the case. Demands to improve the quality of health care are part of a bigger picture, reflecting the changing society in which we live.[4] These demands are not unique to the National Health Service in Britain – most countries are struggling with similar issues and some have been doing so for considerably longer than the UK.

The forces pressing for improved quality in general practice are irresistible. These forces include demands by the public, the media and politicians for greater accountability of public services, the rise of consumerism and the desire for a true partnership between the users of health care and those who provide it. These demands are supported by a trend towards reduced professional power and a fall in implicit trust in health professionals' ability to regulate their own standards. These societal changes are fuelled by unease resulting from media coverage of high profile disasters in the NHS and recognition that there are some systematic problems with the quality of a service that was previously taken for granted.

The public, politicians and professional bodies are now asking for evidence that acceptable standards of care are being delivered by those who work in the NHS. They are also demanding a commitment to continuously improving the quality of care provided. The government is driving change aligned to a strategic plan described in a series of White Papers[5-7] and outlined in the recent NHS Plan.[8] In the following section we consider the kinds of approaches to quality improvement that primary care professionals could use to address these demands.

What approaches are available to improve quality?

There are many different ways of improving quality in primary care. Many of these approaches are already an accepted part of daily practice (Box 1.3). The current focus on quality, through clinical governance, professional revalidation and NHS reappraisal, is helping to bring these together and to adopt a more critical view of the best balance between the approaches for any specific individual, group or for any particular quality improvement task. *Personal Learning Plans* and *Practice Development Plans*[9] are strategic tools to help focus attention on individual and practice needs and rationalise the choice of the most effective improvement methods.

Increasingly these methods recognise the need to assess or measure quality, in order to get a baseline before starting improvement and in order to be able to demonstrate change. Clearly there is no automatic link between measurement and improvement and sometimes there has been so much attention to 'where we are' that we have forgotten 'where we are going and how we are going to get there'. Nevertheless, we live in a society that values 'hard measurement' and this is reflected in the move to develop *quality indicators*.

Box 1.3   Approaches available to improve quality

Clinical and organisational audit

Assessment of user/care experience or satisfaction

Significant event analysis

Lectures, seminars and courses

Reading journals, reviews, books

Assessment by peers

Learning diaries

Development and use of guidelines, risk management and care pathways

---

What are quality indicators?

Quality indicators are specific and measurable elements of practice that can be used to assess the quality of care. They are usually derived from retrospective reviews of medical records or routine information sources. Some authorities differentiate 'quality' from 'activity' or 'performance' indicators. The important issue is that a good quality indicator should define care that is attributable and within the control of the person who is delivering the care. Quality indicators are different from *guidelines*, which are statements of good practice, often loosely defined, that can be used prospectively to guide care. Quality indicators are also different from *standards*, as described in Box 1.4 and outlined in the following section.

What role do quality indicators play in quality improvement?

Quality indicators are easily misused. It is important to recognise that they are *indicators*, rather than definitive judgements about quality. There is no such thing as a perfect quality indicator and it would be inappropriate to apply all indicators in a

---

Box 1.4   An example illustrating the difference between a guideline, an indicator and a standard

---

When managing a patient who is found to have a raised blood pressure recording:

Guideline: if a blood pressure recording is raised on one occasion, the patient should be followed up

Indicator: patients with a blood pressure of greater than 160/90 mmHg should have their blood pressure remeasured within 3 months

Standard: 90% of the patients in the practice with a blood pressure of greater than 160/90 mmHg should have had their blood pressure remeasured within 3 months

---

mechanical way to the care provided for all patients. It is important to set realistic standards for individual indicators, rather than to assume that all care should aim for, or achieve, 100% success on all indicators.

For example an indicator might state that all patients with a blood pressure of greater than 160/90 mmHg should have their blood pressure remeasured within 3 months (Box 1.4). There are good reasons why this might not be possible or desirable: patients might not want to come to surgery or might decide that they have other priorities in their lives; the practice might be in the middle of an influenza epidemic so routine follow-up of other problems is delayed; or the practice nurse or general practitioner might dismiss a 'one-off' reading on the basis of their personal knowledge of the patient. To account for this, it is quite reasonable for practices to set their own standards for specific indicators. For example a well-organised practice might aim for 90% of patients with hypertension to achieve good control, or a practice with a large, mobile population might aim for 65% of eligible patients having a cervical smear. The standards will vary for condition and for practice and are most appropriately set at a local level. The important issue is that standards are reviewed at regular intervals and that there is a commitment to continuously trying to achieve higher standards of care.

The benefit of quality indicators comes from the debate associated with the results: what is an acceptable standard? Why is our care apparently improving or deteriorating? Why are we achieving better/worse levels of care than our neighbouring practices? Protected time to discuss the results and educational support to ensure that indicators are used effectively are essential components of the process. The benefits and problems of using quality indicators to assess and improve quality in general practice are summarised in Boxes 1.5 and 1.6. The debate among health professionals has tended to concentrate on the problems and the negative consequences of using quality indicators. This is hardly surprising given the nature of the indicators in common use and the abuse of comparative data by some parties. However, more sophisticated methods are now being used to develop quality indicators and greater attention is being given to the scientific properties of the resultant indicators. This should result in the future in a more balanced debate about the risks and benefits. This issue is addressed in more detail in Chapter 22.

Box 1.5 The benefits of using quality indicators

Quality indicators can:

Allow comparisons to be made between practices, over time or against gold standards. These comparisons can stimulate and motivate change

Facilitate an objective evaluation of a quality improvement initiative

Be used to ensure accountability and identify unacceptable performance

Stimulate informed debate about quality of care and level of resources

Focus attention on the quality of information in general practice

Help target resources to areas of greatest need

Be quicker and cheaper tools for quality assessment than other tools, e.g. peer review

Inform purchasing decisions and planning of service agreements

---

Box 1.6 The problems of using quality indicators

Quality indicators may:

Encourage a fragmented approach to an holistic and integrated discipline

Assess only easily measurable aspects of care and fail to encompass the more subjective aspects of general practice

Be based on dubious quality data and information that is difficult to access

Be difficult to interpret; for example, apparent differences in care may relate more to random variation, case mix or case severity, rather than real differences in the quality of care

Be expensive and time consuming to produce; the cost–benefit ratio of measuring quality of care is largely unknown

Encourage a blame culture and discourage internal professional motivation

Lead organisations to focus on measured aspects of care to the detriment of other areas and to concentrate on the short term rather than adopting a long-term strategic approach

Erode public trust and professional morale if deficiencies in the quality of care are highlighted

Encourage massaging or manipulation of the data by health professionals or organisations if the results of indicators are published

---

The following chapter describes the methods used to develop the quality indicators

References

1. Donabedian A. *Explorations in quality assessment and monitoring 1*. The definition of quality and approaches to its assessment. Ann Arbor: Health Administration Press, 1980
2. Campbell SM, Roland MO, Buetow S. Defining quality of care. Social Science and Medicine 2000; 51: 1611–1625
3. Seddon ME, Marshall MN, Campbell SM, Roland MO. Systematic review of studies of quality of clinical care in general practice in the United Kingdom, Australia and New Zealand. Accepted for publication in Quality in Health Care 2001
4. Marshall MN. Time to go public on performance? British Journal of General Practice 1999; 49: 691–692
5. Department of Health. A first class service, quality in the NHS. London: Department of Health, 1998
6. NHS Executive. The NHS Performance Assessment Framework, 1999
7. NHS Executive. Quality and Performance in the NHS: High Level Performance Indicators and Clinical Indicators, 1999
8. Department of Health. The NHS plan: a plan for investment, a plan for reform. London: Department of Health, 2000
9. Rughani A. The GP's guide to personal development plans. Oxon: Radcliffe Medical Press, 2000

▶2

Developing the quality indicator set

Stephen Campbell and Jenny Hacker

Key points

▶ Many aspects of general practice are not, and probably can never be, supported by evidence derived from randomised controlled trials.

▶ In order to assess the quality of general practice care it is necessary to combine, in a systematic and rigorous way, the scientific evidence that is available with the opinions and experience of experts.

▶ This chapter describes in detail the six stages of this approach that we used to develop a set of quality indicators for the most common issues presenting to British general practice.

▶ The resulting quality indicators have a high degree of face validity as measures of quality in general practice but require further clinical testing before more definitive judgements about quality can be made.

Methods of developing quality indicators

Quality indicators have been developed in a variety of different ways. The first and most common way has been for a group of people to sit down together around a table and come up with suggestions. These are usually based on readily available information, such as referral rates. This approach has the advantages of speed and simplicity but the disadvantage that resulting indicators may be meaningless to those who want to use them to improve the quality of clinical care.

A second approach is to base indicators purely on published evidence from randomised controlled trials. This 'evidence-based' approach[1] has the advantage of producing rigorous and scientifically acceptable indicators but has two main disadvantages. First, it focuses on a very limited part of general practice, since so much of what is regarded as good quality care in general practice does not have (and probably never will have) experimental evidence to support it. Second, some people have questioned the applicability to individual patients of evidence derived from scientific trials on selected populations.

In response to this, we adopted a third approach, developed over 25 years ago by the RAND Corporation in California.[2] This approach recognises the importance of scientific evidence but is concerned with the application of this evidence to real clinical practice and with the significant gaps in the evidence applicable to some areas of practice. We therefore chose this method of combining scientific evidence with expert opinion in an attempt to produce a more comprehensive and useful set of quality indicators for British general practice. The method has been used extensively in both the USA and the UK, and in both primary and secondary care.[3-8] Despite some criticisms,[9,10] it is generally regarded as the most rigorous and systematic way of combining expert opinion and scientific evidence.[11] Some of the key characteristics of the RAND appropriateness method are summarised in Box 2.1.

Box 2.1   Some of the key characteristics of the RAND appropriateness method [2,7]

Timeliness: produces indicators within a relatively short time period
Systematic: based on a systematic and comprehensive synthesis of available evidence
Knowledge based: builds on the scientific literature by incorporating expert opinion
Quantitative: provides a quantitative measure of the scientific properties of the quality measure

---

The development of the indicators

Researchers from the RAND Health Program have used their appropriateness method to develop primary care quality indicators for over 70 conditions presenting to US primary care physicians.[12-15] On reviewing these indicators it was clear that the structural and cultural differences between the US and UK health systems would result in significant problems if these indicators were applied directly to British general practice. We therefore used a modification of the RAND appropriateness method to adapt the US indicators and develop new indicators that could be used for quality assessment in the UK. The process was undertaken in six stages (Box 2.2):

Box 2.2   Summary of stages in the development of the indicators

1. *Selection of conditions:* 19 common conditions were chosen for which indicators would be developed
2. *Developing the literature reviews and preliminary sets of indicators:* literature reviews were commissioned for each of the conditions and preliminary indicators were developed
3. *Selection of expert panels:* experts in general practice were invited to join panels for a two-stage process to rate the indicators
4. *First-round postal survey:* draft indicators and literature reviews were sent to the panel members, who were asked to rate them in terms of their validity and the importance of recording the data
5. *Second-round panel meetings:* the first-round scores were analysed and the results given back to panellists for a second round of scoring in a 2-day face-to-face panel meeting
6. *Second-round data analysis and drafting of final indicator set:* the second-round scores were used to select only those indicators rated highly for validity and for necessity to record the information on which the indicator was based

---

Stage 1: selection of conditions

We chose to develop quality indicators for the most common clinical conditions presenting to UK general practice, based on the most recent National Morbidity Survey in General Practice.[16] The 19 selected conditions, all of which had been reviewed as part of the RAND project, provide examples of acute, chronic and preventive care and we estimate that they represent about 60% of consultations in UK general practice.

Stage 2: developing the literature reviews and preliminary sets of indicators

The literature reviews are an important part of the indicator development process because they encourage the experts to relate their opinions and experience to the available scientific evidence. New evidence-based reviews (Chs 3–21) were therefore commissioned from leading primary care researchers in the UK. They are not formal systematic reviews but represent comprehensive summaries of the available national and international literature, focusing specifically on evidence directly relevant to general practice in the UK.

At the same time as reviewing the literature, the reviewers were asked to propose a preliminary set of quality indicators for their condition. This set was based on the evidence, national guidelines and professional statements, and was influenced by the indicators developed by the RAND team. The indicator set and supporting data were presented to the expert panels in a structured format. An example is presented in Table 2.1.

Table 2.1 Example of suggested indicator

	Indicator	*Quality of evidence	References	Benefits/ summary
1.2	Patients with coronary artery disease should be advised to take aspirin at a dose of 75–150 mg/day (continued indefinitely) unless they have a contraindication	I	Yusuf et al., 1988; ATC, 1994; Khunti et al., 1999	Absolute reduction in vascular events of about 5%

*Quality of evidence
I   based on evidence from randomised controlled trials
II–1 based on evidence from non-randomised controlled trials
II–2 based on evidence from cohort or case studies
II–3 based on evidence from multiple time series
III   based on opinion or descriptive studies

Stage 3: selection of expert panels

Panels of experts were then convened to rate the preliminary indicators. The definition of an 'expert' in general practice is difficult. We wanted to ensure that the expert panel members were familiar with critical appraisal of scientific evidence but were grounded in the reality of 'real' (though high quality) general practice. We therefore decided to select panel members from the database of Fellows by Assessment of the Royal College of General Practitioners (FBAs), since this award, based on rigorous self- and peer practice-based assessment, is generally regarded as the highest explicit standard attained by service general practitioners. All 196 FBAs in the UK in 1999 were invited to participate. Eighty-two percent responded and 91% of these agreed to take part. Panel members were selected to represent the genders, different types of practice and geographical location and levels of clinical experience. Two panels, each with 9 members, were formed. Each panel was allocated approximately half of the conditions to assess, as summarised in Box 2.3.

Box 2.3 Selected conditions by panel

Panel A	*Panel B*
Coronary artery disease	Asthma
Hypertension	Depression
Diabetes mellitus	Osteoarthritis
Allergic rhinitis	Upper respiratory tract infections
Headache	Acute otitis media
Urinary tract infection	Diarrhoeal disease in children
Dyspepsia	Acne
Cervical screening	Low back pain
Immunisation	Family planning
	Hormone replacement therapy

Stage 4: first-round postal survey

Panel members were sent, by post, the literature reviews and preliminary indicator sets for the conditions being rated by their panel. They were asked to rate all the indicators for their validity as indicators of quality and whether the information was important to be included in the patient's record ('necessity to record'). Each indicator was rated on a 9-point continuous scale for validity and necessity to record, where 1 represented the lowest and 9 the highest rating.

The panellists were advised that an indicator should be considered valid if the following criteria were met:

▶ there was adequate scientific evidence and professional consensus to support it

▶ there were identifiable health benefits to patients who received the care specified by the indicator

▶ panel members considered that doctors or nurses with higher rates of adherence to the indicator would be judged as providing a higher quality service

▶ most factors determining adherence to the indicator were within the control of the doctor or nurse.

The panellists were told that ratings of 1–3 would mean that the indicator was not a valid measure of quality, 4–6 would mean that the indicator was of uncertain or equivocal validity and 7–9 would mean that it was considered to be a valid measure of quality.

An indicator would be considered as necessary to record if the following criteria were met:

▶ failure to document the information could be judged itself to be a marker for poor quality

▶ estimates of adherence to the indicator based on medical record data are likely to be reliable and unbiased.

The panellists were told that a rating of 1–3 would mean that the data should not have to be recorded in the patient's medical record; 4–6 would mean that there is legitimate uncertainty about the need to record the data and 7–9 would mean that the information should be recorded in the patient's notes.

The panellists were also invited to suggest changes to the wording of the indicator if they thought appropriate. An example of a panellist's rating for one indicator is shown in Table 2.2.

Table 2.2 Example of a first-round postal rating

Indicator	Validity	Necessity to record
3.6 All diabetic patients should have an annual fundal examination	1 2 3 4 5 6 7 8 ⑨	1 2 3 4 ⑤ 6 7 8 9

Stage 5: second-round panel meetings

Completed first-round questionnaires were returned by all panellists to the research team. For the second round the ratings were summarised and fed back to the panel members in a face-to-face meeting. The purpose of the meeting was to discuss the first-round ratings, prior to repeating the rating process. No indicators were dropped between rounds, irrespective of how they were rated in round 1, in order to allow panellists the opportunity to discuss each indicator at the panel meeting. The panel meetings lasted for 2 days and were chaired by members of the research team. The chair's role was to facilitate discussion, focusing on the indicators for which there was wide variation in the ratings of different panellists. The panel members were not forced to reach consensus and were encouraged to rate as they saw fit after the discussion for each indicator.

The data were presented to the panellists as an anonymised overall distribution of the first-round scores for all members, together with an individualised first round score for each of the panel members. An example of the feedback and modification (shown in italics) to the indicator is shown in Table 2.3. This shows the rating scale (1–9), the overall distribution of all panel members' scores in italics (i.e. 6 members gave a rating of 3 for validity) and this individual panel member's personal rating in bold (i.e. a validity score of 8 in this example).

Table 2.3   Example of feedback to panel members for second-round ratings

Indicator	Validity		Necessity to record
10.8 Short-acting β₂ agonist should be prescribed for symptomatic relief on an 'as required' basis *unless contraindicated or intolerant*	*1 1 6* 1 2 3 4 5 6 7 8 9	*1*	*3 6* 1 2 3 4 5 6 7 8 9

Stage 6: second-round data analysis and drafting of final indicator set

Only second-round ratings were used to select the final set of indicators. The decision to select or reject indicators was based on their median validity and 'necessity to record' scores and the level of agreement between the scores of panel members.

To be included in the final set, an indicator needed an overall median rating of greater than 7 for validity and greater than 6 for necessity to record, without disagreement within the panel. The RAND research team used greater than 6 for validity and greater than 4 for recording but we chose to use more rigorous cut-off points, influenced in part by our clinical judgement about the final set of indicators. Disagreement was defined in statistical terms as being when 3 or more of the 9 ratings for any 1 indicator were in the 1–3 region and three or more in the 7–9 region.

The number and proportion of indicators rated by the panels as good measures of quality, by condition, is shown in Table 2.4. A higher proportion of indicators for chronic and preventive care were rated valid than for acute care. This highlights the difficulty with making explicit judgements about quality for some aspects of general practice, particularly those that have a weaker evidence base.

Table 2.4   Proportion of indicators rated valid by condition

Condition	Number of indicators rated	Number rated valid	% rated valid
Asthma	29	25	86.2
Family planning and contraception	7	6	85.7
Cervical screening	11	8	72.7
Coronary heart disease	18	13	72.2
Dyspepsia and peptic ulcer disease	13	9	69.2
Acne	9	6	66.7
Hypertension	43	28	65.1
Immunisations	31	20	64.5
Acute otitis media	5	3	60.0
Urinary tract infection	32	19	59.4
Depression	46	25	54.4
Diabetes mellitus	29	15	51.7
Hormone replacement therapy	18	9	50.0
Acute diarrhoeal disease in children	25	11	44.0
Allergic rhinitis	10	4	40.0
Headache	37	11	29.7
Upper respiratory tract infection	27	8	29.6
Osteoarthritis	23	6	26.1
Acute low back pain	22	3	13.6

Further development of the indicator set

A total of 229 indicators for the 19 conditions were rated as valid measures of quality by the expert panels. However, this is just the first step in the process of indicator development. At the end of the panel process the indicators are conceptually valid measures of quality based on systematically combining scientific evidence and expert opinion. The next stage is to test the indicators in clinical settings in order to investigate their scientific properties – factors such as the availability of data in different types of practice, the reliability of data collection, the sensitivity of the indicators to changes in quality and their validity as compared to other measures of quality.

Preliminary field testing has already taken place as part of a demonstration project being conducted by the National Primary Care Research and Development Centre in two localities in England. This has resulted in the removal of some indicators from the set and minor modification to others. However, further evaluation is required in a range of different practices and primary care organisations across the UK in order to determine the usefulness of the indicators at a local level. We would not expect all of the indicators to be usable in all circumstances and, as with all quality indicators, we would encourage an appropriately critical appraisal of the results arising from their use.

The following 19 chapters describe the evidence base for each of the clinical conditions for which the indicators were developed and presents a list of the indicators for each condition.

References

1. McColl A, Roderick P, Gabbay J, Smith H, Moore M. Performance indicators for primary care groups: an evidence based approach. BMJ 1998; 317: 1354–1360
2. Brook RH, Chassin MR, Fink A, Solomon DH, Kosekoff J, Park RE. A method for the detailed assessment of the appropriateness of medical technologies. International Journal of Technology Assessment in Health Care 1986; 2: 53–63
3. Kahan JP, Bernstein SJ, Leape LL, Hilborne LH, Park RE, Parker L et al. Measuring the necessity of medical procedures. Medical Care 1994; 32, 357–365
4. Leape LL, Hilborne LH, Schwartz JS et al. The appropriateness of coronary artery bypass graft surgery in academic medical centres. Annals of Internal Medicine 1996; 125: 8–18
5. Gray D, Hampton JR, Bernstein SJ, Kosecoff J, Brook RH. Audit of coronary angiography and bypass surgery. Lancet 1990; 335: 1317–1320
6. Scott EA, Black N. Appropriateness of cholecystectomy in the United Kingdom – a consensus panel approach. Gut 1991; 32: 1066–1070
7. Shekelle PG, Kahan JP, Bernstein SJ, Leape LL, Kamberg CJ, Park RE. The reproducibility of a method to identify the overuse and underuse of procedures. New England Journal of Medicine 1998; 338: 1888–1895
8. Campbell SM, Roland MO, Shekelle PG, Cantrill JA, Buetow SA, Cragg DK. The development of review criteria for assessing the quality of management of stable angina, adult asthma and non insulin dependent diabetes mellitus in general practice. Quality in Health Care 1999; 8: 6–15
9. Kassirer JP. The quality of care and the quality of measuring it. New England Journal of Medicine 1993; 329, 1263–1264
10. Hicks NR. Some observations on attempts to measure appropriateness of care. British Medical Journal 1994; 309: 730–733
11. Naylor D. What is appropriate care? (editorial). New England Journal of Medicine 1998; 338: 1918–1920
12. Kerr EA, Asch S, Hamilton EG, McGlynn EA. Quality of care for general medical conditions: a review of the literature and quality indicators. Santa Monica, CA: RAND Health Program, 1998

13. Kerr EA, Asch S, Hamilton EG, McGlynn EA. Quality of care for cardiopulmonary conditions: a review of the literature and quality indicators. Santa Monica, CA: RAND Health Program, 1998

14. McGlynn EA, Kerr EA, Damberg C, Asch S. Quality of care for women: a review of selected clinical conditions and quality indicators. Santa Monica, CA: RAND Health Program, 1997

15. McGlynn EA, Asch SM. Developing a Clinical Performance Measure. American Journal of Preventive Medicine (RAND Health Program Reprint Service 98–9Q) 1998;14

16. McCormick A, Fleming A, Charlton J. Morbidity statistics from general practice: 4th National Study 1991–1992. London: OPCS, DH, RCGP, 1995

▶3

Asthma

Stephen Campbell

Importance

Estimating the prevalence of asthma in the UK is difficult, largely because of varying definitions and diagnostic criteria. However, most estimates suggest that approximately 3.4 million people in the UK have asthma;[1,2] corresponding to 6% of children and 3–4% of adults.[3] Asthma is frequently underdiagnosed in elderly people because of the wide differential diagnosis.[4] A general practitioner will see, on average, 85 asthmatic patients per year, each of whom makes an average of 3 consultations.[5] The consultation rate for asthma doubled between 1981–2 and 1991–2 and the prevalence of asthma is increasing.[1,6]

Asthma as a cause of death is uncommon: 1459 deaths in the UK in 1995.[1] However, asthma places a huge burden on society. There were 93 870 hospital admissions for asthma in 1994–5 with an average length of stay of 3.5 days. The total cost per annum to the UK is estimated at £2000 million per year.[1] For example, the cost to the NHS of childhood asthma alone was estimated at between £79 million and £135 million in 1990.[3] The value of lost productivity for work days in 1994/95 was estimated at £1139 million.[6] The net ingredient cost of asthma prescriptions was estimated at £511 million in 1995–6.[1] The financial cost of primary care consultations relating to asthma is approximately £60 million per annum.[1] Moreover, 90% of people with asthma feel that it has an impact on their lives,[7,8] particularly sleep disturbance and activity limitation.[1] Over one-third of children with asthma miss at least a week of school per year because of asthma symptoms.[2]

This review focuses upon quality indicators for the management of asthma in primary care in the UK for both children and adults. There is a lack of evidence to back up many routine management procedures. Moreover, many systematic reviews on asthma contain methodological flaws.[9] Evidence, where it exists, relates mostly to the efficacy of medication.[5,10,11] In 1999 the Royal College of Physicians organised a seminar to discuss measuring clinical outcomes in asthma.[6] This seminar concluded that a set of common aims and standards are needed for UK general practice. There is some evidence that the British Thoracic Society (BTS) guidelines, while widely disseminated, are not widely used.[12]

Review of evidence relating to indicator set

Screening

There is no evidence to support screening for asthma in asymptomatic patients. However, there has been some debate about the importance of general practices keeping an asthma register and using it to audit asthma care.[4]

Diagnosis

Correct diagnosis of asthma is important. There is some overlap between asthma and chronic obstructive pulmonary disease, for which recent guidelines have been published,[13] but asthma is usually best seen in isolation. Asthma is a chronic inflammatory disorder characterised by breathing difficulties caused by narrowing of the airways (bronchi) of the lung. It is a hypersensitive response to the exposure of precipitating factors such as allergens (i.e. pollen or house dust), irritants, cold air, drugs, viral infections or exercise. Onset may occur at any age but is most common in childhood: it is the most common chronic disease in children. The condition may be seasonal and is prone to acute exacerbations.

An initial diagnosis of asthma is based largely on presenting signs and symptoms. Symptoms include wheezing, shortness of breath, cough (including nocturnal cough), chest tightness and (yellow) sputum production. The diagnosis is confirmed by finding 15% or greater reversibility in response to β_2 agonists or a diurnal variability in peak flow of at least 15%. A single, isolated peak flow reading should not be used to diagnose asthma. Diagnosis of asthma in children under the age of 5 years, especially those aged 0–2 years, is dependent upon symptoms rather than lung function tests.[4]

The diagnosis should therefore be based on a detailed medical history, including possible precipitating factors, peak flow variability, recurrent symptoms and response to medication. In order to facilitate effective management, the diagnosis of asthma, and current medication, should be prominently displayed and easily identifiable in the medical record (indicator 1).

Treatment

The goals of asthma management are to keep patients well on the minimum possible medication and at a reduced risk of attack. Treatment includes both pharmacological and non-pharmacological strategies.

Patient education/management

Patients with asthma should be offered education/advice about their condition and management, including recognising danger signs, seeking medical advice early in an attack, avoiding precipitating factors and the importance of compliance with treatment. Many published studies tend to combine different educational interventions, making it difficult to identify which are the most important. Limited patient education, particularly simple provision of information, does not appear to improve health outcomes.[14] However, structured patient education is beneficial,[4] especially if intensive. For example, education that includes self-monitoring by either

PEF or symptoms can improve knowledge, patient outcomes/morbidity and beneficially alter behaviour.[5,15]

There is no evidence to support all adult patients with asthma receiving a self-management or written action plan.[5] However, patients on high-dose steroids or who have been hospitalised should be given a self-management plan, detailing the appropriate response to changes in peak flow and symptoms.[15,16] (indicator 2).

There is no evidence to support the routine use of allergen immunotherapy in primary care,[5,17] nor sole treatment with yoga, acupuncture or homeopathy.[5,18] There is little evidence to support routine influenza vaccination of all asthmatics, though vaccination can reduce mortality during epidemics.[19]

Peak flow

Measurement of peak flow is regarded as an integral part of asthma management. However, there is no evidence to suggest that routine self-managed monitoring of peak flow should be mandatory for all patients because it does not alter patient outcomes. In addition, it may be misleading because large morning dips can represent transient rather than long-term poor control. However, recordings of normal and predicted peak flow act as a baseline for ongoing management and may suggest a need for change in management. There is some consensus, based on opinion rather than evidence, that peak flow should be recorded annually in all patients who can use a peak flow meter.[4,5,15] However, asthma can be seasonal and many asthmatics are not seen every year.

As a compromise, the expert panels recommended that patients on current maintenance medication for asthma, and those not on current medication but who have presented with asthma symptoms in the last 5 years, should have had their normal and predicted peak flow measured at least once in the last 5 years (indicators 3–6).

Smoking

While there is no evidence linking the recording of smoking status with improved outcomes, the smoking status of all asthmatics should be asked and recorded at least once every 5 years[5,15] (indicator 7). This applies to all asthmatics aged 13 and over as the prevalence of smoking in teenagers is high. Smoking should be strongly discouraged in all asthmatics. Smokers should be advised to stop, using a combination of advice and support from a health professional[5] and nicotine replacement therapy in those motivated to quit[5,15].

Inhalers and devices

Inhaler technique should be checked at least once every 5 years to ensure that patients can use their devices properly[5,15] (indicator 8). Inhaler technique should be checked whenever an increase in maintenance therapy is being considered to ensure that poorly controlled symptoms cannot be explained by poor inhaler technique. Drug delivery devices should be tailored to individual patients according to adequacy/ease of use, patient compliance and patient preference.[5,15,20]

Level of control of symptoms

Assessing and monitoring the level of control of symptoms has been strongly recommended.[6,15,21] This should apply to every consultation where the primary presenting problem is asthma. All patients on current medication, and/or those who have presented with asthma in the last 5 years, should be asked about daily, nocturnal and activity-limiting symptoms (indicator 9).

Pharmacological therapy

Current medication should be displayed prominently and recorded in the notes (indicator 1) as this facilitates subsequent management. The medication regime should be determined by BTS guidelines[4] but specific prescribing decisions should be tailored to individual circumstances.[5]

Patients with asthma should not be prescribed a beta-blocker as beta-blockade promotes airway reactivity[15] (indicator 10). Data from an ongoing study at National Primary Care Research and Development Centre (NPCRDC) suggests that 0.7% of adult asthmatics from a sample of over 1000 are prescribed beta-blockers.

If patients have exercise-induced asthma, short-acting β_2 agonist should be prescribed for use before exercise.[5,15]

Mild asthma (step 1 BTS)

Short-acting β_2 agonists are effective bronchodilators.[5] There is no evidence suggesting any therapeutic value from regular use of short-acting β_2 agonists. Rather, all patients should be prescribed a short-acting β_2 agonist on an 'as required' basis for symptomatic relief[5] (indicator 11) and advised to use the minimum daily dose necessary to control their symptoms.[4] There are no clinically important differences between different short-acting β_2 agonist inhalers and as such the cheapest viable preparation should be used for all patients. However, inhaled drugs are more efficacious for children than bronchodilator syrups.[4] Ipratropium bromide may be more efficacious than salbutamol in children under the age of 12 months as first-line medication.[4]

Moderate asthma (steps 2–3 BTS)

In patients whose symptoms are not controlled by occasional use of relief bronchodilators, for example those experiencing daily or nocturnal symptoms or a falling peak flow, prophylactic medication is indicated. This should begin with low-dose anti-inflammatory agents (step 2). Beclomethasone, Budesonide 100–400 µg twice daily or Fluticasone 50–200 µg twice daily are most frequently prescribed; in patients who are intolerant of or refuse steroids, cromoglycate or nedocromil may be used. Most authorities recommend that patients over 5 years of age should be prescribed an anti-inflammatory drug if they are using their short-acting β_2 agonist more than once a day (indicator 12). Others have suggested that use more than 2 or 3 times per day is more realistic.[4,5,15] Use of β-agonists as a quality indicator is not recommended.[6]

Severe asthma (BTS steps 4–5 for adults and schoolchildren; step 4 for children under 5)

Data from the NPCRDC suggests that 72% of adult asthmatics are managed at BTS step 1 or 2 and 11% at step 3. For all patients with severe asthma, adults and children, routine management requires flexible prescribing tailored to the needs of individual patients.[4,5]

Exacerbations

Patients consulting with an acute exacerbation of asthma should have a peak flow taken and recorded[5,15] as this enables an assessment of severity compared to baseline/predicted PEF and helps to determine immediate and subsequent management (indicator 13).

In acute situations requiring immediate bronchodilator therapy, pulse rate and respiratory rate should be assessed and recorded[4,15] (indicator 14). If peak flow is taken during an exacerbation for uncontrolled or acute asthma treated with nebulised β_2 agonist, then peak flow should be repeated 15–30 minutes after treatment.[4,5,15]

There is no established protocol for admitting a patient to hospital based on peak flow during an exacerbation. The British Thoracic Society guidelines suggest that while there is some evidence for a figure of 33% of predicted/best peak flow, 50% is more widely accepted.[4] If patients are not admitted to hospital and are treated within primary care for an exacerbation, they should be treated with oral corticosteroids[4,10,15] if their PEF is <50% of predicted/best (indicator 15).

Oral corticosteroids should be prescribed for adults at a dose of 30–40 mg/day until symptoms have resolved: for at least 7 days[5,10] but possibly for up to 21 days.[4,15] Oral corticosteroids can be stopped from full dosage after an exacerbation; a reducing course after treatment of less than 2 weeks duration is not necessary.[5]

Referral

There is little evidence about the benefits of referral of patients with asthma, either from primary to secondary care or between health care professionals within primary care. Recommendations regarding referral are taken from the British Thoracic Society guidelines.[4] Patients should be referred to hospital for a specialist opinion if they are suspected to have occupational asthma,[5,15] if they have been prescribed or are being considered for oral steroids as maintenance therapy,[5,15] or if nebulisers are used in, or being considered for, maintenance therapy[15] (indicator 16).

Overview of data sources used in this review

This review is based on the 1997 British Thoracic Society Guidelines on Asthma Management (BTS),[4] published evidence based review criteria for adult asthma[15] and the updated 1999 North of England guideline for the evidence based primary care management of asthma in adults.[3] Several Cochrane reviews were also consulted[10,11,14,17,18,20,23] as well as two recent reports on clinical outcomes in asthma.[6,21] In addition a search was conducted on the electronic database MEDLINE using the key words: asthma + general practice + UK, up to July 2000.

Acknowledgements

I would like to thank Professor Sean Hilton, St George's Hospital Medical School, for his helpful comments on this chapter.

Recommended quality indicators for asthma

Diagnosis

1.   a. A diagnosis of asthma should be easily identifiable in the notes
    b. Current medication should be recorded in the notes

Management

2. Written self-management plans should be offered to all adults with asthma who:
   1. are on high-dose inhaled steroids
   2. have been hospitalised with asthma
3. Patients with asthma, if on medication, should have their normal peak flow measured on at least one occasion
4. Patients presenting with asthma in the last 5 years but not on current medication should have their normal peak flow measured on at least one occasion
5. Patients with asthma, if on current medication, should have their predicted peak flow calculated on at least one occasion
6. Patients presenting with asthma in the last 5 years but not on current medication should have their predicted peak flow calculated on at least one occasion
7.   a. Patients with asthma over the age of 12 should have been asked about their smoking status within the last 5 years
    b. Patients with asthma over the age of 10 should have been given smoking advice
    c. Smokers should be advised how to stop, using a combination of advice and support from a health professional
8. Patients on current medication or presenting with asthma should have their inhaler technique checked at least once every 5 years
9. For patients on current medication or presenting with asthma, patients should be asked at every asthma consultation in the last year about
    a. any difficulty sleeping due to asthma
    b. any asthma symptoms during the day, i.e. cough, wheeze
    c. whether asthma has interfered with usual daily activities
10. Patients with asthma should not have been prescribed a beta-blocker unless there is justification for doing so
11. Short-acting β_2 agonist should only be prescribed on an 'as required' basis
12. Patients using short-acting β_2 agonist more than once per day should be offered prophylactic medication tailored to their individual needs
13. Patients consulting with an acute exacerbation of asthma should have a PEF taken and this should be compared to their normal or predicted PEF
14. In acute situations requiring emergency treatment the following should be assessed and recorded:
    a. pulse rate
    b. respiratory rate
15. Patients with an exacerbation should be treated with oral corticosteroids by the GP, unless contraindicated or intolerant, if their PEF is <50% of normal/predicted unless they are admitted to hospital

Referral

16. Patients should be referred to a specialist if they have:
    a. occupational asthma
    b. been prescribed, or are being considered for, oral steroids as maintenance therapy
    c. been prescribed or are being considered for nebulisers in maintenance therapy

Further reading

For a review of the current knowledge base for the management of asthma in the UK, the North of England Evidence Based Guideline[5] and the revised British Thoracic Society guideline[4] provide a comprehensive starting point. The Royal College of Physicians report 'Measuring clinical outcome in asthma: a patient centred approach'[6] provides a good summary of current thinking in terms of measuring clinically important outcomes in asthma. Price and Ryan, *Asthma: The Key Facts*, offers a useful general text.[2]

References

1. National Asthma Campaign. National Asthma Audit 1999/2000. London: National Asthma Campaign, 1999
2. Price DB, Ryan D. Asthma: the key facts. Middlesex: Allen & Hanburys, 1998
3. Lenney W, Wells NEJ, O'Neill BA. The burden of paediatric asthma. European Respiratory Review 1994; 4: 49–62
4. British Thoracic Society. Guidelines on the management of asthma. Thorax 1997; 52: S1-S21
5. The primary care management of asthma in adults. North of England Evidence Based Guideline. Centre for Health Services Research, University of Newcastle-upon-Tyne, 1999. Available at: http://www.ncl.ac.uk/chsr/publicn/tools/asthma_s.htm
6. Royal College of Physicians. Measuring patient outcome in asthma. A patient-focused approach. London: Royal College of Physicians, 1999
7. Osman LM, Calder C, Robertson R, Friend JA, Legge JS, Douglas JG. Symptoms, quality of life, and health service contact among young adults with mild asthma. American Journal of Respiratory Critical Care Medicine 2000; 161: 498–503
8. Nocon A, Booth T. The social impact of asthma. Family Practice 1991; 8: 37–41
9. Jadad AR, Moher M, Bowman GP, Booker L, Sigouin C, Fuentes M, Stevens R. Systematic reviews and meta-analyses on treatment of asthma: critical evaluation. British Medical Journal 2000; 320: 537–540
10. Rowe BH, Spooner CH, Ducharme FM, Bretzlaff JA, Bota GW. Corticosteroids for preventing relapse following acute exacerbations of asthma. The Cochrane Library 1999, issue 3
11. Plotnick LH, Ducharme FM. Combined inhaled anticholinergics and β_2 agonists for initial treatment of acute paediatric asthma. The Cochrane Library 1999, issue 3
12. Roghmann MC, Sexton M. Adherence to asthma guidelines in general practices. Journal of Asthma 1999; 36: 381–387
13. Culpitt SV, Rogers DF. Evaluation of current pharmacotherapy of chronic obstructive pulmonary disease. Opin Pharmacother 2000; 1: 1007–1020
14. Gibson PG, Coughlan J, Wilson AJ et al. Limited patient education programs for adults with asthma. The Cochrane Library 1999, issue 3
15. Campbell SM, Roland MO, Shekelle PG, Cantrill JA, Buetow SA, Cragg DK. The development of review criteria for assessing the quality of management of stable angina, adult asthma and non insulin dependent diabetes mellitus in general practice. Quality in Health Care 1999; 8: 6–15
16. Thoonen BP, Jones KP, van Rooij HA, van den Hout AC, Smeele I, Grol R, van Schayck CP. Self-treatment of asthma: possibilities and perspectives from the practitioner's point of view. Family Practice 1999; 16: 117–122
17. Hammarquist C, Burr ML, Gotzsche PC. House dust mite control measures for asthma. The Cochrane Library 1999, issue 3
18. Linde K, Jobst K, Panton J. Acupuncture for chronic asthma. The Cochrane Library 1999, issue 3
19. Ahmed AE, Nicholson KG, Nguyen van Tam J. Reduction in mortality associated with influenza vaccine during 1989–1990 epidemic. Lancet 1995; 346:
20. Cates. Holding chambers versus nebulisers for beta-agonist treatment of acute asthma. The Cochrane Library 1999, issue 3
21. Pearson M, Goldacre M, Coles J et al. (eds). Health outcome indicators: asthma. Report of a working group to the Department of Health. Oxford: National Centre for Health Outcomes Development, 1999
22. Campbell SM. Measuring quality of care in general practice (QUASAR study). NPCRDC Annual Report, 2000
23. Abramson MJ, Puy RM, Weiner JM. Allergen immunotherapy for asthma. The Cochrane Library 1999, issue 3

4

Coronary heart disease

Nicholas Hicks, Tim Lancaster and David Mant

Importance

Coronary heart disease (CHD) is the leading cause of death in the UK. More than one-third of the population die from atherosclerosis and 1 in 12 men dies from CHD before the age of 65. People are at varying risk from CHD depending upon a number of risk factors, including age, gender, family history, smoking, hypertension, dyslipidaemia and diabetes mellitus. The absolute risk of dying of CHD can be predicted from these risk factors.

The importance of CHD and the potential to reduce the associated morbidity and mortality has been recognised by the launch of the CHD National Service Framework. The framework focuses resources first on those with established CHD (myocardial infarction or angina; secondary prevention), then those at high risk but without established disease (primary prevention).

Review of evidence relating to quality indicator set

Acute cardiac pain and unstable angina

Aspirin

Patients presenting with symptoms of acute myocardial infarction or unstable angina should receive 300 mg of aspirin immediately and before hospital admission (indicator 2). This is supported by a large body of experimental evidence.[1-5] The standard preparations of aspirin in the UK are 75 mg and 300 mg. The Antiplatelet Triallists Collaboration (ATC) overview data[5] show that aspirin started immediately and continued for 1 month reduces vascular events (myocardial infarction, stroke or vascular death) by 29% (95% CI 65–77%). The number needed to treat (NNT) to prevent 1 vascular death is 26. Prasad et al.[6] showed administration of aspirin before admission in only 169 (65%) of cases (based on 260 GP hospital referrals of patients with chest pain in Glasgow).

Delay

When a patient reports symptoms suggestive of myocardial infarction an ambulance should be called immediately (before attending the patient).[7,8] In one study[7] (based on 2213 patients aged <75 years with evolving myocardial infarction admitted to 4 district general hospitals in the UK), the estimated number of deaths prevented by reducing delay from onset of symptoms to admission to 1 hour or less was 86/1000 patients. Another study[8] showed an increased odds of survival (2.3, 95% CI 1.5–3.6) if patients were attended before admission by a defibrillator-capable emergency medical service; the benefit was maximal if the patient was seen within 11 minutes of reporting symptoms. It would be possible to set a standard for delay. To minimise case fatality, the delay from symptom presentation to attendance by staff equipped with defibrillator equipment should be less than 11 minutes and the delay to hospital admission and administration of fibrinolytic therapy should be less than 1 hour. Despite the strong evidence, the feasibility of attaining this standard would be influenced by geographical context and therefore we have not included it as a quality indicator.

Chronic stable angina and post-infarct care

The effective management of CHD requires an up-to-date disease register (indicator 1).

Aspirin

Patients with coronary artery disease (CAD) should be advised to take aspirin at a dose of 75–150 mg/day (continued indefinitely) unless they have a contraindication (indicator 2).[5,9–11] The ATC overview data[5] show that among 400 patients randomised in 7 trials comparing antiplatelet therapy with controls there was an absolute reduction in vascular events of about 5%. The Khunti paper[11] shows that the proportion of patients with a contraindication to aspirin is about 10% and that effective feedback and audit can increase levels of acceptance of treatment by post-myocardial infarction patients without contraindications in UK general practice to 97% (95% CI 95–98%). In the UK aspirin may well be purchased directly from pharmacies rather than prescribed; however, the recommendation to take aspirin will normally be recorded in the patient's medical record.

Blood pressure

All patients with CAD should have their blood pressure measured at least every 5 years (indicator 3, evidence adapted by panel); those with a systolic blood pressure ≥150 mmHg or a diastolic blood pressure ≥90 mmHg should be monitored at least yearly (indicator 4). All patients with CAD and a mean systolic blood pressure ≥160 mmHg or a mean diastolic blood pressure ≥100 mmHg should be given dietary advice and anti-hypertensive medication as necessary aiming to attain a mean blood pressure of ≤140/85 (indicators 5 and 6).[12,13] The Collins & Peto overview[12] of 4 large and 13 small randomised trials showed that a reduction of 5–6 mmHg in blood pressure sustained over 5 years reduces coronary events by 16% and stroke by 38%. The Hansson et al. (HOT) trial[13] showed that the lowest risk of cardiovascular events occurred with a mean diastolic blood pressure achieved of 82.6 mmHg. However, the absolute gains were small provided blood pressure was less than 150/90 mmHg (the audit standard).

Cholesterol

If a patient has established CAD, his or her blood lipids should be measured and dietary advice and lipid-lowering therapy given where necessary to achieve a total cholesterol level of at least <5mmol/L (LDL ≤3 mmol/L; indicators 7, 8).[14-18] The Scandinavian Simvastatin Survival Study Group trial[14] showed that among patients aged 35–70 years with angina or previous myocardial infarction and a total cholesterol between 5.5 and 8.0 mmol/L, simvastatin reduced risk of death by 30% (95% CI 15–42%) over 5 years. The Tang review[18] showed that dietary interventions in free living subjects can also reduce cholesterol, but the reduction achieved is much less than with statin treatment (5% at 12 months compared with 20–30%). Following the principle that prescription of statins should be driven by levels of absolute risk rather than threshold lipid values, it is likely that increasing numbers of patients with established CAD will receive this treatment irrespective of their initial cholesterol level, so the target of cholesterol <5 mmol/L should be regarded as the minimum standard in this population.

Smoking

All patients with established CAD should have their smoking status recorded in their medical record (indicator 9). All smokers should be given smoking cessation advice by their doctor and this should also be documented (indicator 10).[19-22] The British doctors' study by Doll and Peto[19] reported 25 years ago that after 9 years of smoking cessation the CVD risk of ex-smokers approximates the risk of lifelong non-smokers. A recent Cochrane review[22] shows that advice by physicians, reinforced by written information and nicotine replacement therapy where appropriate, is effective in helping people to stop smoking. The odds of cessation following brief advice versus no advice (based on 18 studies) is 1.7 (95% CI 1.5, 2.0) which approximates to an absolute difference in cessation rate of 3%.

ACE inhibition and beta blockade

All patients with a history of acute myocardial infarction should be given a beta-blocking drug indefinitely, unless specific contraindications exist (indicator 11). ACE inhibitor drugs should be considered in all patients, and should always be given if there is documented evidence of impaired systolic function and no specific contraindication (indicator 12).[23-26] The AIRE extension study[24] confirmed a relative mortality reduction of 36% (95% CI 15–52%) in those treated with ramipril for 1 year. The absolute reduction in deaths was 6% at 2 years (NNT 17) and 11% at 5 years (NNT 9). In CIBIS-II[25] all-cause mortality was 12% in the placebo group and 17% in the intervention group – a relative mortality reduction of 34% (95% CI 19–46%). In the Freemantle et al. overview,[26] the mortality reduction in long-term trials was 23% (95% CI 15–31%). There is good reason to argue that left ventricular function should be assessed to decide on optimal therapy for all patients with a history of myocardial infarction. Lack of open access to echocardiography stopped us from recommending this as a quality standard in UK general practice.

Blood sugar

Blood sugar should be measured in all patients with CAD or suspected CAD to assess overall risk of vascular death and to guide management of other risk factors (indicator 13).[13,27,28] The Haffner et al. study[27] confirms the greatly increased CHD mortality risk of patients with CAD and hyperglycaemia. The UK Prospective Diabetes Study[28] shows that CHD risk in diabetics is not closely correlated with the degree of glycaemic control, but that risk is significantly reduced by effective treatment of high blood pressure. The Hanssen et al. (HOT) trial[13] showed a 51% reduction in major cardiovascular events in patients with diabetes mellitus in target group $\leq$80 mmHg compared with target group $\leq$90 mmHg.

Recommended quality indicators for coronary heart disease

Diagnosis

1 The diagnosis of CAD should be clearly identifiable on the electronic or paper records of all known CAD patients

Treatment

2 Patients with CAD should be advised at least once to take aspirin at a dose of 75–150 mg/day (continued indefinitely) unless they have a contraindication

3 Patients with CAD should have their blood pressure measured and documented at least every 2 years

4 Patients with CAD should have their blood pressure checked at least yearly if they have a systolic blood pressure $\geq$140 mmHg and/or diastolic blood pressure $\geq$85 mmHg

5 Patients with CAD and a sustained systolic blood pressure $\geq$160 mmHg or a diastolic blood pressure $\geq$100 mmHg should be offered antihypertensive medication (as necessary to attain a mean blood pressure of $\leq$140/85)

6 Patients with CAD and hypertension on treatment and a mean systolic blood pressure of >150/90 should be offered a change in therapy (if not changed in the previous 6 months)

7 Patients with established CAD should have had their blood lipids measured within the last 5 years

8 Patients with established CAD with a total cholesterol level of >5 mmol/L should be offered dietary advice or lipid lowering therapy or a change in therapy (if not changed in the prior 6 months)

9 Patients with established CAD should have their smoking status recorded since their disease has been diagnosed

10 Smokers should be given smoking cessation advice at least once since diagnosis

11 Patients with a history of acute myocardial infarction should be currently prescribed a beta-blocking drug indefinitely, unless specific contraindications exist

12 ACE inhibitors should be currently prescribed for all patients for whom there is documented evidence of impaired systolic function and no specific contraindications or intolerance documented in the records

13 Patients with CAD should have their blood sugar measured once since diagnosis

---

Overview of data sources used in this review

The authors did not carry out a new comprehensive literature review of CHD care for this chapter as this had very recently been carried out as a step in the development of the national service framework. The working group was fortunate in having one of the main scientific contributors to the service framework (NH) among its membership.

Further reading

Department of Health. National Service Framework for Coronary Heart Disease. London: Department of Health, 2000.

References

1. ISIS-2 Collaborative Study Group. Randomised trial of intravenous streptokinase, oral aspirin, both or neither among 17187 cases of suspected acute MI: ISIS-2. Lancet 1987; 1: 349–360
2. Theroux P, Ouimet H, McCans J et al. Aspirin, heparin or both to treat acute unstable angina. New England Journal of Medicine 1988; 319: 1105–1111
3. RISC group. Risk of MI and death during treatment with low dose aspirin and IV heparin in men with unstable coronary disease. Lancet 1990; 336: 827–830
4. Yusuf S, Sleight P, Help P, McMahon S Routine medical management of acute MI: lessons from overviews of recent randomised controlled trials. Circulation 1990; 82 (suppl): 117–134
5. Antiplatelet Trialists Collaboration. Collaborative overview of RCTs of antiplatelet therapy. British Medical Journal 1994; 308: 81–106
6. Prasad N, Srikanth S, Wright A, Dunn F. Management of suspected MI before admission: updated audit. British Medical Journal 1998; 316: 353
7. Norris R, Wong P, Dixon G et al. Effect of time of onset to coming under care on fatality of patients with acute MI. Heart 1998; 80: 114–120
8. Nichol G, Stiell I, Laupacis A. Cumulative meta-analysis of the effectiveness of defibrillator-capable emergency medical services for victims of out-of-hospital cardiac arrest. Annals of Emergency Medicine 1999; 34: 517–525
9. Yusuf S, Wittes J, Friedman L. Overview of results of randomised controlled trials in heart disease. Journal of the American Medical Association 1988; 260: 2259–2263
10. Krumholz H, Radford M, Ellerbeck E et al. Aspirin for secondary prevention after acute MI in the elderly: prescribed use and outcomes.
11. Khunti K, Sorrie R, Jennings S, Farooqi A. Improving aspirin prophylaxis after MI in primary care. British Medical Journal 199; 319: 297
12. Collins R, Peto R. Anti-hypertensive drug therapy: effects on stroke and coronary heart disease. In: Swales J. Textbook of hypertension. Oxford: Blackwell, 1994: 1156–1164
13. Hansson L, Zanchetti A, Carruthers S et al. Effects of intensive blood pressure lowering and low dose aspirin in patients with hypertension. Lancet 1998; 351: 1755–1762
14. Scandinavian Simvastatin Survival Study Group. RCT of cholesterol lowering in 4444 patients with coronary heart disease. Lancet 1994; 344: 1383–1389
15. Miettinen T, Pyorala K, Olsson A et al. Cholesterol lowering therapy in women and elderly patients with MI or angina pectoris: findings from 4S study. Circulation 1997: 96(12): 4211–4218
16. LIPID study group. Prevention of CV events and deaths with pravastatin in patients with CHD. New England Journal of Medicine 1998; 339: 1349–1357
17. Lewis S, Moye L, Sacks F et al. Results of the cholesterol and recurrent events (CARE) trial. Annals of Internal Medicine 1998; 129; 681–689
18. Tang J, Armitage J, Lancaster T et al. Systematic review of dietary intervention to lower total blood cholesterol in free living subjects. British Medical Journal 1998; 316; 1239
19. Doll R, Peto R. Mortality in relation to smoking: 20 years observation on male British doctors. British Medical Journal 1976; 2: 1525–1536
20. Hermannson B, Omenn G, Kronmal R. Beneficial six-year outcome of smoking cessation in older men and women with CAD: results from the CASS registry. New England Journal of Medicine 1988; 24: 1365–1369
21. Cavender J, Rogers W, Fisher L. Effects of smoking on survival and morbidity in the coronary artery surgery study (CASS) J: 10 year follow-up. American Journal of Cardiology 1992; 20: 287–294
22. Silagy C, Ketteridge S. Physician advice for smoking cessation. Cochrane Review (last updated January 1999)
23. Hennekens CH, Albert CM, Godfried SL et al. Adjunctive drug therapy of acute MI from the clinical trials. New England Journal of Medicine 1996: 335: 1660–1667
24. Hall A, Murray G, Ball S. Follow-up study of patients randomly allocated to ramipril or placebo for heart failure after acute MI (AIRE extension study). Lancet 1997; 349: 1493–1497
25. Dargie H, Lechat P. Cardiac Insufficiency Bisoprolol Study II (CIBIS–II): a randomised trial. Lancet 1999; 353: 9–13
26. Freemantle N, Cleland J, Young P et al. B-blockade after MI: systematic review. British Medical Journal 1999; 318: 1730–1737

27. Haffner SM, Lehto S, Ronnemaa T et al. Mortality from CHD in subjects with type 2 diabetes and in non-diabetic subjects with and without prior MI. New England Journal of Medicine 1998; 339: 2289–2234

28. UK Prospective Diabetes Study Group. Tight blood pressure control and risk of microvascular and macrovascular complications in hypertensive type 2 diabetes. British Medical Journal 1998: 317: 703–713

▶ 5

Depression

Tony Kendrick

Importance

In UK general practice roughly 5% of attenders are found to be suffering from major depression, 5% from minor depression, and around 15% from some depressive symptoms.[1] Depression accounts for around one-third of days lost from work due to ill health in the UK,[2] and around 1 in 5 general practice consultations.[3] Kind & Sorenson[4] estimated the direct costs of treating depression in the UK in the early 1990s to be around £400 million, and the indirect costs, including mortality costs and lost productivity, at £3000 million.

Review of evidence relating to indicator set

Screening and prevention

Studies of patients attending UK practices have shown that half of those with depression go unrecognised by their doctors.[5,6] Many of these patients are consulting with physical symptoms, which may explain this lack of recognition. Depression may also be recognised but not recorded,[7] because of the stigma attached to the diagnosis, or its implications for insurance risks or difficulties obtaining employment. Using questionnaires to screen for depression cannot be recommended, however, as the natural history of the disorder is not well described, and it has not been convincingly demonstrated that identifying cases through questionnaires leads to an improved outcome.[8] It is likely that recognition leads to a better outcome only if it is followed by adequate treatment, which often is not the case.[9]

Older depressed women should be screened for unidentified hypothyroidism, which is present in around 1 in 10 women over the age of 50 and can present as depression[10] (indicator 1). Depression is strongly associated with female gender,[11,12] lower socioeconomic status,[13,14] poverty[15] unemployment,[14,16] separation or divorce[13,17] and poor housing.[18] Predisposing factors among women include demanding childcare and poor social support.[19] Therefore GPs and other members of primary care teams should ask about symptoms of depression among patients presenting with any of these risk factors.

Diagnosis

The diagnosis of major depressive disorder is based primarily on DSM-IV (Diagnostic and Statistical Manual, 4th version) criteria in the USA,[20] and the ICD-10 (World Health Organization's International Classification of Diseases, 10th edition) criteria are very similar.[21] The criteria state that at least five of the following nine symptoms must be present in a two-week period to receive a diagnosis of major depression: depressed mood; markedly diminished interest or pleasure in almost all activities; fatigue; insomnia/hypersomnia; significant weight loss/gain; psychomotor agitation/retardation; feelings of worthlessness or guilt; impaired concentration; recurrent thoughts of death or suicide.

One of the symptoms must be depressed mood or loss of interest in usual activities. The symptoms should be present most of the day, nearly daily, for a minimum of two weeks, and accompanied by significant impairment of functioning. Primary care versions of both DSM-IV and ICD-10 classifications have been developed, which essentially adopt the same criteria for major depression. Two symptoms that are commonly presented in primary care have relatively high positive predictive value for the presence of depression, namely sleep disturbance and fatigue.[22,23] Any patient presenting with one of these symptoms should also be asked about the other seven symptoms (indicator 2).

Associated factors that the doctor should seek out include substance abuse, medications that cause depression, general medical disorders and bereavement[24] (indicator 3).

Suicidal ideas should be sought out routinely in any depressed patient (indicators 4, 5), plus any specific plans to carry it out (e.g. obtaining a weapon, putting affairs in order, making a suicide note).[24] People who have specific plans for suicide should be referred to a psychiatrist urgently and may be admitted to hospital.

Treatment

Drug treatment

Antidepressant medications are recommended as first-line treatments for major depressive disorder, as this form of treatment is likely to be most cost-effective. Drug treatment is advised if patients have enough symptoms for long enough, and impaired functioning, even if there seems to be an understandable cause for depression such as social problems[1,25,26] (indicator 6). This advice is based on a UK primary care study which found that patients with probable major depressive disorder responded to tricyclic antidepressant drug treatment, but those with minor depression did not. There was no difference between those with endogenous and non-endogenous depression, and the authors recommended treatment for probable major depression, regardless of demographic characteristics, past history of depression or endogenous features.[27] Further research is needed, and a placebo-controlled trial is currently being undertaken of the efficacy of selective serotonin reuptake inhibitors (SSRIs) and problem solving for minor depression and dysthymia in a primary care population.[28]

UK guidelines usually recommend tricyclics as first-line treatment, because they are effective and cheaper than newer drugs.[1,26] Amitriptyline at a dose of 125 mg per day is effective in most cases of major depression,[29-31] but titration up to this level may not be possible due to drowsiness and anticholinergic side-effects. Consequently, lower doses are often given, but these may not be superior to placebo.[29,32] SSRIs do not need to be titrated upwards like tricyclics and can be started at a therapeutic dose, but they are more expensive than the older drugs. It has been suggested that they may still be more cost-effective, as their side-effect profile means they may be better tolerated and therefore more effective in preventing costly complications of depression.[25] However, meta-analyses of trials comparing the two groups for their efficacy and discontinuation rates have found no overall difference in efficacy and only small absolute differences (around 3%) in drop-out rates.[33-36] The advantage for SSRIs holds only against the older, more toxic compounds (amitriptyline and imipramine) and not the newer tricyclics or tricyclic-related drugs.[37]

The SSRIs have different side-effect profiles, are less cardiotoxic and safer in overdosage, and so can be recommended as first-line treatment where side-effects are likely to be a problem or where there is a clear suicide risk.[1,25]

A number of antidepressants which are neither tricyclic-related nor SSRIs have been developed more recently, including venlafaxine, mirtazapine, nefazodone and reboxetine. Expert reviews of these newer drugs suggest that they are all as effective as the tricyclic antidepressants and SSRIs, but differ in their side-effect profiles and, being more expensive, can be recommended only as second-choice agents.[38,39] Whatever the choice of drug, it should be prescribed at a therapeutic dose: either the dose range recommended in the *British National Formulary*[40] or a lower dose if the patient has responded to this.

Psychological treatments

Controlled trials of non-directive counselling in general practice have provided little good evidence for its effectiveness, although the studies have often been characterised by small sample sizes, high drop-out rates, short follow-up periods, ill-defined therapies and inadequate evaluation.[41-43] A trial of social work support found significant benefit for women with an acute episode of depression on top of a long-standing depression compared with usual treatment.[44] On the other hand, a comparison of referral for counselling and casework by a social worker compared with routine GP care proved only slightly more effective and considerably more costly.[45]

There is good evidence for the efficacy of cognitive-behavioural therapy and problem solving, compared to usual care.[46] In mild to moderate depression cognitive-behavioural therapy, when given by trained therapists over 15–20 sessions, has been shown to be as effective as antidepressant treatment.[47-49] Moreover, two follow-up studies suggest that it may also prevent relapse,[50,51] although this requires more evaluation. Studies of shorter courses of cognitive therapy are needed, as this may be more cost-effective.

Problem solving has been developed in UK primary care as a 6-session structured treatment and can be delivered by primary care professionals after a short training period.[52,53] The combination of problem solving with antidepressant medication was found to be no more effective than either treatment alone.[54] The effectiveness of psychodynamic therapies has not been convincingly demonstrated in primary or secondary care.[55-57]

If the patient is referred for psychological treatment, the treatment should be one that has been shown to be effective (indicator 6). At the time of writing this review and the time that the expert panels were conducted, proven effective therapies available in UK primary care were cognitive-behavioural treatment and problem solving. Since this time, a new trial has been published which suggests that non-directive counselling may be as effective as cognitive-behavioural treatment.[58] Referral for psychological treatment is indicated if the depression is mild to moderate, medication is unsuitable or the patient declines it, the depression seems closely related to interpersonal or social problems or the patient requests psychological treatment.

Medication should be considered if there is no response to psychological treatment at 6 weeks, or only partial response at 12 weeks.

Follow-up

The patient should be seen within the first 2–4 weeks after prescribing antidepressant drug treatment, as this is the time when the drug is beginning to work, plus side-effects may need to be discussed and adherence encouraged (indicator 7). Patients who respond to medication should be continued at the same dose for 4–9 months after they have recovered, to avoid early relapse[1,24-26,59,60] (indicator 8).

It has been shown that adherence in the first few weeks is improved by the following instructions;[61] antidepressants should be taken for 2–4 weeks before a noticeable effect; the medication should be taken daily and continued even if feeling better; it should not be stopped without checking with the doctor; side-effects should be explained by the doctor. It is particularly important to emphasise to patients that antidepressants are not addictive, as this misconception is held by more than 85% of the UK public.[62]

The UK guidelines do not make specific recommendations about follow-up intervals but every 4 weeks once treatment is established would be a reasonable recommendation.[1,23] If the patient shows no response to the medication by 6 weeks, then the clinician might consider changing to a second antidepressant.[63] If the second medication fails to resolve the patient's symptoms, referral to a consultant psychiatrist is indicated[63] (indicator 9).

A randomised trial of referral for specialist treatment for patients with major depression showed only small clinical advantages over routine general practitioner care, but specialist treatment cost at least twice as much.[45] Routine referral of all patients with major depression to a psychiatrist or psychologist is therefore unlikely to be cost-effective in the UK and cannot be recommended on current evidence. However, referral is recommended in the UK consensus guidelines[1] in the following circumstances (indicator 9): where there is uncertainty about the diagnosis, e.g. a possible psychosis; consultation for management, e.g. failure to respond to initial treatment; for hospital investigations, e.g. a brain scan to check for organic disease; suicidal or violent behaviour or serious self-neglect; coexisting problems such as substance misuse or eating disorder; occasionally as a result of pressure from the patient or others; and occasionally to reinforce the general practitioner's advice.

Maintenance treatment is designed to prevent new episodes of depression. Patients should be considered for maintenance treatment if they have had 3 or more episodes of major depressive disorder, or 2 episodes plus another circumstance (family history of bipolar disorder, history of recurrence within 1 year, family history of recurrent major depression, onset before age 20 or severe life-threatening episodes). Most studies of longer-term treatment for the prevention of recurrence have shown benefit from all classes of antidepressants, with relapse rates of around 20% compared to 40% on placebo.[59,64] However, the benefit of long-term drug treatment has been shown only in secondary care among patients with major depression and the same benefits may not apply in primary care.[64] The choice usually depends on what has produced acute benefit in the particular patient. The decision about maintenance will also depend on the severity of the episodes, their impact on the person's life and career, and the person's willingness to commit him- or herself to long-term treatment.[60] A psychiatric opinion may be valuable in deciding whether or not to continue treatment.

Elderly people

Risk factors for depression in elderly people, which should prompt enquiry about depressive symptoms, include living alone, caring for a disabled relative, bereavement and early dementia.[64-67] As many as 40–50% of elderly people in nursing or residential care homes will be found to be suffering from depression.[68] Around one-third of widowed elderly people will meet DSM criteria for major depression 2 months after the loss, one-quarter 2–7 months after, and 15% 3 months after[69] (indicator 10).

Several chronic illnesses including diabetes, osteoarthritis, chronic obstructive pulmonary disease, Parkinson's disease, chronic back pain and multiple unexplained somatic complaints, are also associated with depression.[70] The US AHCPR guidelines[24] recommend that patients with a cerebrovascular accident, myocardial infarction, dementia, malignancy or chronic pain should be asked about symptoms of depression, as a high proportion will be depressed (indicator 11).

Older people are at greater risk of adverse reactions to antidepressants, in particular to the tricyclics, due to concurrent illness, interactions with other medicines, altered pharmacokinetics and forgetfulness.[71,72] Reviews of controlled studies of SSRIs have suggested that they are as efficacious for the treatment of depression in elderly people, although almost all the studies cited were on relatively physically healthy outpatients.[73,74] Theoretically, SSRIs should be better tolerated by older people, because of their relative lack of anticholinergic and antihistaminergic effects, and of adverse effects on cognition, seizure threshold and the cardiovascular system.[75,76] However, a UK review of drop-out rates in trials comparing tricyclic antidepressants and SSRIs in the elderly pointed out that they have not demonstrated any consistent advantage for SSRIs.[71] SSRIs also have side-effects, including inhibition of cytochrome oxidase P450 2D6, so concomitant prescription may potentiate other drugs including benzodiazepines and antihistamines.[74]

As with the younger age group, the SSRIs seem to have advantages over the older tertiary amine tricyclics, but no apparent advantage over newer tricyclic-related drugs. Two recent meta-analyses showed no differences between heterocyclic and serotonergic antidepressants in efficacy or tolerability.[77,78] For the reasons given above,

Recommended quality indicators for depression

Screening
1. Women over 50 with depressive symptoms should have been screened for hypothyroidism in the last 3 years
2. For any patient presenting with sleep disturbance or fatigue enquiry should be made about other symptoms of depression (e.g. depressed mood, markedly diminished interest or pleasure in almost all activities, significant weight loss/gain, psychomotor agitation/retardation, fatigue, feelings of worthlessness (guilt), impaired concentration and recurrent thoughts of death or suicide)

Diagnosis
3. In the assessment of depression, enquiry should be made about:
   a. alcohol use
   b. substance misuse
   c. current medication
4. The presence or absence of suicidal ideas should be sought out routinely in all patients found to be depressed
5. Patients with suicidal thoughts should be asked if they have specific plans to carry out suicide

Treatment
6. Patients with a diagnosis of depressive disorder (low mood or lack of interest in usual activities for 2 weeks plus 4 of 7 other symptoms and impaired functioning) should be offered an effective first-line treatment (antidepressant or cognitive-behavioural therapy or problem solving)
7. Patients with depression prescribed antidepressant drug treatment should be invited for review by a health care professional within 4 weeks of initiating antidepressant drug treatment
8. Treatment with an antidepressant should be continued for at least 4 months after recovery from depression
9. Patients with depression should be referred for a specialist opinion where there is evidence of :
   a. a possible psychosis
   b. organic brain disease
   c. the patient exhibiting suicidal behaviour
   d. serious self-neglect
   e. violent behaviour
   f. non-response to two antidepresants

The elderly
10. GPs should ask about the presence or absence of symptoms of depression among people aged 65 and over who have been bereaved in the last 12 months
11. GPs should ask about the presence or absence of symptoms of depression among people aged 65 and over who are suffering from:
    a. a recent cerebrovascular accident
    b. malignancy (except for skin cancer)
    c. early dementia
    d. Parkinson's disease
    e. Huntington's disease
    f. Chronic pain
    g. Multiple unexplained symptoms
12. Antidepressant treatment should be initiated at half the usual starting dose in patients aged 75 and over

it is not possible to be prescriptive about the choice of drug for elderly patients, as this will depend on a number of factors, including previous history of tolerance of, and response to, a particular drug, possible interactions with concurrent drugs and concurrent physical illness. Whichever drug is used, a consistent recommendation in the literature is to start with lower doses, whether of tricyclics (e.g. initially 10–25 mg once daily of amitriptyline instead of 25–50 mg) or SSRIs (e.g. 10 mg instead of 20 mg of fluoxetine)[74] (indicator 12). Uncontrolled studies have suggested that drug treatment is beneficial for major depression persisting for more than 6 months after bereavement, but randomised controlled trials need to be carried out to confirm this benefit.[79]

Overview of data sources used in this review

This review is based on work from the following sources: the 1992 UK expert conference consensus statement; the 1993 British Association for Psycho-pharmacology guidelines; the 1993 Effective Healthcare Bulletin from the Centre for Health Economics, University of York; and the 1999 North of England Evidence-based Guideline Development Project guidelines for the choice of antidepressants in primary care and the US AHCPR depression guidelines. In addition, selected review articles and original research papers identified through an electronic search of the Cochrane, Embase and Medline databases up to December 1999 were accessed, together with hand searching of other papers identified from the reference lists of papers found electronically.

Further reading

Paykel ES, Priest RG. Recognition and management of depression in general practice: consensus statement. British Medical Journal 1992; 305: 1198–1202

Montgomery SA. Guidelines for treating depressive illness with antidepressants. Journal of Psychopharmacology 1993; 19–23

School of Public Health, University of Leeds, Centre for Health Economics, University of York, and Research Unit, Royal College of Physicians. Effective Health Care Bulletin: The treatment of depression in primary care. York: Department of Health, 1993

Eccles M, Freemantle N, Mason J. North of England Evidence-based Guideline Development Project: Summary version of guidelines for the choice of antidepressants for depression in primary care. Family Practice 1999; 16: 103–111

References

1. Paykel ES, Priest RG. Recognition and management of depression in general practice: consensus statement. British Medical Journal 1992; 305: 1198–1202
2. Jenkins R. Minor psychiatric disorder in employed young men and women and its contribution to sickness absence. British Journal of Industrial Medicine 1985; 42: 147–154
3. Williams P, Tarnopolsky A, Hand D, Shepherd M. Minor psychiatric morbidity and general practice consultations: the West London Survey. Psychological Medicine 1986 (Monograph suppl 9): 1–37
4. Kind P, Sorensen J. The costs of depression. International Clinical Psychopharmacology 1993; 7: 191–195
5. Goldberg DP, Blackwell B. Psychiatric illness in general practice. A detailed study using a new method of case identification. British Medical Journal 1970; 2: 439–443
6. Freeling P, Rao BM, Paykel ES, Sireling LI, Burton RH. Unrecognised depression in general practice. British Medical Journal 1985; 290: 1880–1883
7. Rost KG, Smith GR, Guise B, Matthews D. The deliberate misdiagnosis of major depression in primary care. Archives of Family Medicine 1994; 3: 333–337
8. Wright AF. Should general practitioners be testing for depression? British Journal of General Practice 1994; 44: 132–135

9. Goldberg D, Privett M, Ustun B, Simon G, Linden M. The effects of detection and treatment on the outcome of major depression in primary care: a naturalistic study in 15 cities. British Journal of General Practice 1998; 48: 1840–1844

10. Hodkinson H, Denham M. Thyroid function tests in the elderly in the community. Age and Ageing 1977; 6: 67–70

11. Blazer DG, Kessler RC, McGonagle K, Swartz M. The prevalence and distribution of major depression in a national community sample: The National Comorbidity Survey. American Journal of Psychiatry 1994; 151: 979–986

12. Kessler RC, McGonagle K, Zhao S et al. Lifetime and 12-month prevalence of DSM-III-R psychiatric disorders in the United States. Archives of General Psychiatry 1994; 51: 8–19

13. Regier DA, Farmer ME, Rae DS et al. One-month prevalence of mental disorders in the United States and sociodemographic characteristics: the Epidemiologic Catchment Area Study. Acta Psychiatrica Scandinavica 1993; 88: 35–47

14. Weich S, Lewis G. Poverty, unemployment, and common mental disorders: population based cohort study. British Medical Journal 1998; 317: 115–119

15. Bruce M, Takeuchi DT, Leaf PJ. Poverty and psychiatric status: longitudinal evidence from the New Haven epidemiologic catchment area study. Archives of General Psychiatry 1991; 48: 470–474

16. Kessler RC, Turner JB, House J. Intervening processes in the relationship between unemployment and health. Psychological Medicine 1987; 17: 949–961

17. Romans SE, Walton VA, McNoe B, Herbison GP, Mullen PE. Otago women's health survey 30-month follow-up I: onset patterns of non-psychotic psychiatric disorder. British Journal of Psychiatry 1993; 163: 733–738

18. Platt S, Martin C, Hunt S. The mental health of women with children living in deprived areas of Great Britain: the role of living conditions, poverty and unemployment. In: Goldberg D, Tantam D, eds. The public health impact of mental disorder. Toronto: Hogrefe & Huber, 1990; 124–135

19. Brown GW, Bifulco A, Harris T. Life events, vulnerability and onset of depression: some refinements. British Journal of Psychiatry 1987; 150: 30–42

20. American Psychiatric Association. Substance-related disorders. In: Diagnostic and statistical manual of mental disorders: DSM-IV. Washington, DC: American Psychiatric Association, 1994; 175–205

21. World Health Organization. The ICD-10 classification of mental and behavioural disorders: diagnostic criteria for research. Geneva: World Health Organization, 1993

22. Blacker O, Clare AW. The prevalence and treatment of depression in general practice. Psychopharmacology 1988; 95: S14–S17

23. Gerber PD, Barrett JE, Barrett JA et al. The relationship of presenting physical complaints to depressive symptoms in primary care patients. Journal of General Internal Medicine 1992; 7: 170–173

24. AHCPR Depression Guideline Panel. Depression in primary care: vol. 1. Detection and diagnosis. Clinical practice guideline, no. 5. Rockville, MD: US Department of Health and Human Services, Public Health Service, Agency for Health Care Policy and Research, 1993

25. Montgomery SA. Guidelines for treating depressive illness with antidepressants. Journal of Psychopharmacology 1993; 19–23

26. School of Public Health, University of Leeds, Centre for Health Economics, University of York, and Research Unit, Royal College of Physicians. Effective Health Care Bulletin: The treatment of depression in primary care. York: Department of Health, 1993

27. Paykel ES, Hollyman JA, Freeling P, Sedgwick P. Predictors of therapeutic benefit from amitriptyline in mild depression: a general practice placebo-controlled trial. Journal of Affective Disorders 1988; 14: 83–95

28. Barrett JE, Williams JW, Oxman TE et al. The treatment effectiveness project. A comparison of the effectiveness of paroxetine, problem-solving therapy, and placebo in the treatment of minor depression and dysthymia in primary care patients: background and research plan. General Hospital Psychiatry 1999; 21: 260–273

29. Blashki TG, Mowbray R, Davies B. Controlled trial of amitriptyline in general practice. British Medical Journal 1971; 1: 133–138

30. Thomson J, Rankin H, Ashcroft GW, Yates CM, McQueen JK, Cummings SW. The treatment of depression in general practice: a comparison of L-tryptophan, amitriptyline, and a combination of L-tryptophan and amitriptyline with placebo. Psychological Medicine 1982; 12: 741–751

31. Hollyman JA, Freeling P, Paykel ES et al. Double-blind placebo-controlled trial of amitriptyline among depressed patients in general practice. Journal of the Royal College of General Practitioners 1988; 38: 393–397

32. Thompson C. The prescribing of antidepressants in general practice. II: A placebo-controlled trial of low-dose dothiepin. Human Psychopharmacology 1989; 4: 191–204

33. Song F, Freemantle N, Sheldon TA et al. Selective serotonin reuptake inhibitors: meta-analysis of efficacy and acceptability. British Medical Journal 1993; 306: 683–687
34. Montgomery SA, Henry J, McDonald G et al. Selective serotonin reuptake inhibitors: meta-analysis of discontinuation rates. International Clinical Psychopharmacology 1994; 9: 47–53
35. Anderson IM, Tomenson BM. Treatment disontinuation with selective serotonin reuptake inhibitors compared with tricyclic antidepressants: a meta-analysis. British Medical Journal 1995; 310: 1433–1438
36. Geddes J, Freemantle N, Mason J, Eccles M, Boynton J. SSRIs versus other antidepressants for depressive disorder. Cochrane Library document. Oxford: Cochrane Database of Systematic Reviews, 1999
37. Hotopf M, Hardy R, Lewis G. Discontinuation rates of SSRIs and tricyclic antidepressants: a meta-analysis and investigation of heterogeneity. British Journal of Psychiatry 1997; 170: 120–127
38. Anon. Three new antidepressants. Drug and Therapeutics Bulletin 1996; 34: 65–68
39. Anon. Mirtazapine – another new class of antidepressant. Drug and Therapeutics Bulletin 1999; 37: 1–3
40. British Medical Association, Royal Pharmaceutical Society of Great Britain. British National Formulary. London: BMA & Pharmaceutical Press, 2001
41. Friedli K, King M. Counselling in general practice – a review. Primary Care Psychiatry 1996; 2: 205–216
42. Effective Health Care Bulletin. Mental health promotion in high-risk groups. York, NHS Centre for Reviews and Dissemination, 1997
43. Friedli K, King MB, Lloyd M, Horder J. Randomised controlled assessment of non-directive psychotherapy versus routine general practitioner care. Lancet 1997; 350: 1662–1665
44. Corney RH. The effectiveness of attached social workers in the management of depressed female patients in general practice. Psychological Medicine 1984; 14 (Monograph suppl 6): 1–47
45. Scott A, Freeman C. The Edinburgh primary care depression study: treatment outcome, patient satisfaction and cost after 16 weeks. British Medical Journal 1992; 304: 883–887
46. Brown C, Schulberg HC. The efficacy of psychosocial treatments in primary care: a review of randomized controlled trials. General Hospital Psychiatry 1995; 17: 414–424
47. Teasdale JD, Fennell M, Hibbert GA, Amies P. Cognitive therapy for major depressive disorder in primary care. British Journal of Psychiatry 1984; 144: 400–406
48. Ross M, Scott M. An evaluation of the effectiveness of individual and group cognitive therapy in the treatment of depressed patients in an inner city health centre. Journal of the Royal College of General Practitioners 1985; 35: 239–242
49. Blackburn IM, Bishop S, Glen A, Whalley LJ, Christie JE. The efficacy of cognitive therapy in depression: a treatment trial using cognitive therapy and pharmacotherapy, each alone and in combination. British Journal of Psychiatry 1981; 139: 181–189
50. Blackburn IM, Eunson KM, Bishop S. A two-year naturalistic follow-up of depressed patients treated with cognitive therapy, pharmacotherapy and a combination of both. Journal of Affective Disorders 1986; 10: 67–75
51. Shea MT, Elkin I, Imber SD et al. Course of depressive symptoms over follow-up: findings from the National Institute of Mental Health Treatment of Depression Collaborative Research Programme. Archives of General Psychiatry 1992; 49: 782–787
52. Mynors-Wallis LM, Gath DH, Lloyd-Thomas AR, Tomlinson D. Randomised controlled trial comparing problem solving treatment with amitriptyline and placebo for major depression in primary care. British Medical Journal 1995; 310: 441–445
53. Mynors-Wallis LM, Davies I, Gray A, Barbour F, Gath D. A randomised controlled trial and cost analysis of problem-solving treatment for emotional disorders given by community nurses in primary care. British Journal of Psychiatry 1997; 170: 113–119
54. Mynors-Wallis LM, Gath DH, Day A, Baker F. Randomised controlled trial of problem solving treatment, antidepressant medication, and combined treatment for major depression in primary care. British Medical Journal 2000; 320: 26–30
55. Andrews G. The essential psychotherapies. British Journal of Psychiatry 1993; 162: 447–451
56. Svartberg M, Styles TC. Comparative effects of short-term psychodynamic psychotherapy: a meta-analysis. Journal of Consulting and Clinical Psychology 1991; 59: 7014
57. Crits-Christoph P. The efficacy of brief dynamic psychotherapy: current status and future directions. American Journal of Psychiatry 1992; 149: 151–158
58. Ward E, King M, Lloyd M, Bower P, Sibbald B, Farrelly S. Randomised controlled trial of non-directive counselling, cognitive-behavioural therapy, and usual general practitioner care for patients with depression. I: Clinical effectiveness. British Medical Journal 2000; 321: 1383–1388
59. Montgomery SA. Prophylaxis in recurrent unipolar depression: a new indication for treatment studies. Journal of Psychopharmacology 1989; 3: 47–53
60. Paykel E. Tertiary prevention: longer-term drug treatment in depression. In: Kendrick T, Tylee A, Freeling P, eds. The prevention of mental illness in primary care. Cambridge: Cambridge University Press, 1996: 281–293

61. Lin E, von Korff M, Katon W et al. The role of the primary care physician in patients' adherence to antidepressant therapy. Medical Care 1995; 33: 67–74

62. Priest RG, Vize C, Roberts A, Roberts M, Tylee A. Lay people's attitude to treatment of depression: results of opinion poll for Defeat Depression Campaign just before its launch. British Medical Journal 1996; 313: 858–859

63. AHCPR Depression Guideline Panel. Depression in primary care: vol. 2. Treatment of major depression. Clinical practice guideline, no. 5. Rockville, MD: US Department of Health and Human Services, Public Health Service, Agency for Health Care Policy and Research, 1993

64. Livingston G, Hawkins A, Graham N, Blizard B, Mann A. The Gospel Oak Study: prevalence rates of dementia depression and activity limitation among elderly residents in Inner London. Psychological Medicine 1990; 20: 137–146

65. Iliffe S, Haines A, Gallivan S, Booroff A, Goldenberg E, Morgan P. Assessment of elderly people in general practice. 1. Social circumstances and mental state. British Journal of General Practice 1991; 41: 9–12

66. Iliffe S, Haines A, Stein A, Gallivan S. Assessment of elderly people in general practice. 3. Confiding relationships. British Journal of General Practice 1991; 41: 459–461

67. Iliffe S, See Tai S, Haines A et al. Assessment of elderly people in general practice 4. Depression, functional ability and contact with services. British Journal of General Practice 1993; 43: 371–374

68. Mann A, Graham N, Ashby D. Psychiatric illness in residential homes for the elderly: a survey in one London borough. Age and Ageing 1984; 13: 257–265

69. Zisook S, Schucter S. Depression through the first year after the death of a spouse. American Journal of Psychiatry 1991; 148: 1346–1352

70. Wells KB, Golding JM, Burnam MA. Affective, substance use and anxiety disorders in persons with arthritis, diabetes, heart disease, high blood pressure, or chronic lung conditions. General Hospital Psychiatry 1989; 11: 320–327

71. Livingston MG, Livingston HM. New antidepressants for old people? The evidence that newer drugs are much better than the old is thin. British Medical Journal 1999; 318: 1640–1641

72. Koenig HG, Meador KG, Cohen HG et al. Detection and treatment of major depression in older medically ill hospitalised patients. International Journal of Psychiatry in Medicine 1988; 18: 17–31

73. Menting JE, Honig A, Verhey FR et al. Selective serotonin reuptake inhibitors (SSRIs) in the treatment of elderly depressed patients: a qualitative analysis of the literature on their efficacy and side effects. International Clinical Psychopharmacology 1996; 11: 165–175

74. Newhouse PA. Use of serotonin selective reuptake inhibitors in geriatric depression. Journal of Clinical Psychiatry 1996; 57(suppl 5): 12–22

75. Naranjo CA, Herrmann N, Mittmann N, Bremner KE. Recent advances in geriatric psychopharmacology. Drugs and Aging 1995; 7: 184–202

76. Rothschild AJ. The diagnosis and treatment of late-life depression. Journal of Clinical Psychiatry 1996; 57 (suppl 5): 5–11

77. Mittmann N, Herrmann N, Einarson TR et al. The efficacy, safety and tolerability of antidepressants in late life depression: a meta-analysis. Journal of Affective Disorders 1997; 46: 191–217

78. McCusker J, Cole M, Keller E, Bellavance F, Berard A. Effectiveness of treatments of depression in older ambulatory patients. Archives of Internal Medicine 1998; 158: 705–712

79. Rosenzweig A, Pasternak RE, Prigerson H, Miller MD, Reynolds CF. Bereavement-related depression in the elderly. Is drug treatment justified? Drugs and Aging 1996; 8: 323–328

6

Diabetes mellitus

Adrian Freeman and Michael Hall

Importance

Diabetes mellitus is one of the most common of the endocrine diseases in all populations and all age groups. It is divided into two types: type 1 (traditionally called insulin dependent diabetes mellitus) and type 2 (traditionally called non-insulin dependent diabetes mellitus). Classifications can also include type 3 (e.g. genetically determined types such as MODY, endocrinopathies) and type 4 (gestational diabetes mellitus). A further group (impaired glucose tolerance) has fasting glucose below diabetes diagnostic levels but above the normal range, i.e. 6.1–<7.0 mmol/L.

Over 1 million people in the UK have diabetes, of which the majority have type 2.[1] Diabetes is associated with excess morbidity and mortality. Long-term complications are commonly described as microvascular or macrovascular. Microvascular complications include: retinopathy, which may lead to blindness; nephropathy, which may lead to renal failure; and peripheral neuropathy, which may lead to amputation. Macrovascular complications lead to the increased risk of stroke, myocardial infarction and peripheral vascular disease, all as a consequence of the increased risk of atheroma affecting large vessels. Treatment aims to reduce the morbidity and mortality and allow the patient to maintain a quality of life that is affected as little as possible by the disease.

Review of evidence relating to indicator set

Screening

The National Screening Committee is currently reviewing the evidence and is expected to make recommendations to screen high-risk groups.

Diagnosis

New World Health Organization (WHO) criteria dictate that symptomatic patients with a fasting blood glucose ≥7.0 mmol/L are diabetic[2] and they should therefore have a diagnosis of diabetes mellitus entered on their notes. The diagnostic criteria are more stringent than in the past because many patients with type 2 diabetes have evidence of treatable complications already present at diagnosis.[3] One study modelled existing data regarding HbA1c levels and suggested that a cut-off HbA1c level of 7% for diagnosing diabetes achieved a sensitivity of 99.6% and specificity of 99.9%.[4] Another cross-sectional analysis study identified problems of false-positive diagnosis in those individuals with a fasting blood glucose between 7 and 7.8 mmol/L and suggest that a diagnosis of diabetes should only be made with a fasting blood glucose $\geq$7 mmol/L and a raised HbA1c level. The WHO criteria emphasise that the patient must have symptoms plus a raised single fasting glucose. If there are no symptoms there should be two separate raised fasting blood glucose tests or an abnormal glucose tolerance test before a diagnosis of diabetes is made. These levels are for plasma glucose measured at a laboratory and not whole blood fingerprick tests using a meter. Whole blood fingerprick tests have lower corresponding values; i.e. 7 mmol/L plasma blood glucose is equivalent to 6.1 mmol/L whole blood glucose assuming that the meter is calibrated correctly.

Register

All practices should have a register of diabetic patients and an effective system of recall and review (indicator 1). Several factors have led to an increased role for primary care in the management of diabetes. These include better training of primary care doctors and nurses, easier access for patients, overcrowded hospital clinics and government policy. A Cochrane review looked at randomised trials of hospital versus GP care of diabetics.[5] The reviewers concluded that 'Unstructured care in the community is associated with poorer follow up, greater mortality and worse glycaemic control than hospital care. Computerised central recall with prompting for patients and their family doctors can achieve standards of care as good as or better than hospital outpatient care, at least in the short term. The evidence supports better provision of regular prompted recall and review of people with diabetes by willing general practitioners and demonstrates that this can be achieved, if suitable organisation is in place'. It should be noted that none of the studies in the Cochrane review included children and the majority were for type 2 diabetic patients.

Treatment

Education
All diabetics should receive education about their condition and its management, particularly the dietary aspects. A meta-analysis has shown that educational intervention in adults with diabetes results in an improvement in patient knowledge, weight loss, dietary compliance, psychological outcomes and glycosylated haemoglobin levels.[6]

Glycaemic control
For all patients with diabetes, achieving good glycaemic control is important (indicators 2 and 3). An HbA1c level as close as possible to 7.0% should be the target. It is usually recommended that HbA1c levels should be checked at least annually, though there is no trial evidence to support this recommendation. In order to maintain best glycaemic control more frequent testing may be needed for some patients. However, because of the nature of the test, there is no point in testing more often than every 3 months. It is usually assumed that laboratories in the UK are now standardised

for HbA1c estimations, but in fact assay levels vary; the levels stated assume that the normal HbA1c is <6.1%.

Improved control of blood glucose has delayed the development and progression of retinopathy, nephropathy and neuropathy in patients with type 1 diabetes (DCCT)[7] and those with type 2 diabetes (UKPDS).[8] The UKPDS study achieved a median HbA1c of 7% in the intervention group as compared to a median of 7.9% in the control group. Similarly the DCCT trial achieved HbA1c levels of around 7% through intensive insulin treatment. The UKPDS exclusion criteria included: MI in the previous year; current angina; heart failure; more than one vascular event; serum creatinine greater than 175 mmol/L; retinopathy requiring laser treatment; severe concurrent illness; and inadequate understanding. As a consequence, of 7616 patients originally referred 5102 were actually recruited into the study. In addition, the study enrolled patients at diagnosis and, as the authors acknowledge, HbA1c increases progressively over time whatever the intervention. UKPDS data show a continuous relationship between the risks of microvascular complications and glycaemia, such that for every percentage point decrease in HbA1c (e.g. 9–8%) there was a 35% reduction in the risk of complications.

Data from general practice suggests that the actual level of control achieved is considerably higher than the level recommended by experts.[9]

Type 1 diabetes
All type 1 diabetic patients will need insulin.

Type 2 diabetes
Traditionally treatment of this group has been on a scale of intervention starting with diet alone then, if control is poor, moving onto oral hypoglycaemics and finally insulin treatment if necessary. In the UKPDS study[8] only 58% of the total person years in the control group were spent on diet alone before hyperglycaemia led to the need for additional therapy. Similarly in the intervention group it was difficult to maintain control on monotherapy and additional therapies were usually required.

Blood pressure
Diabetic patients should have their blood pressure controlled to a level of <140/85 mmHg (indicators 4.1 and 4.2). Hypertension increases the already high risk of cardiovascular disease associated with diabetes. One systematic review on antihypertensive treatment in diabetes analysed individual patient data for 5823 people with diabetes within 14 randomised controlled trials.[10] The authors concluded that primary intervention trials indicated a treatment benefit for cardiovascular disease, but not for all-cause mortality in people with diabetes. For secondary prevention there was an improvement in all-cause mortality in diabetic subjects.

The subsequent UKPDS study demonstrated that control to these levels in type 2 diabetes reduced the risk of any non-fatal or fatal diabetic complications.[11] Antihypertensive therapy was compared between an ACE inhibitor and a beta-blocker. Both were equally effective and both achieved the same outcomes with no significant differences in microalbuminuria or proteinuria. A recently published study suggests that there may be a class effect from ACE inhibitors in diabetes, which is independent of the blood pressure lowering effect.[12]

Feet
Feet should be examined for abnormalities such as ulcers, reduced vibration sense and reduced or absent peripheral pulses (indicators 5.1 and 5.2). If there is any evidence of foot deformities, history of foot ulceration or significant vascular or neuropathic disease then the patient should be referred to a foot care clinic (or equivalent) for education, chiropody and protective shoes. Fifteen percent of people with diabetes develop foot ulcers associated with peripheral neuropathy and/or ischaemia.[13] For people with healed diabetic foot ulcers the 5-year cumulative recurrence rate is 66% and the amputation rate is 12%.[14] Foot ulcers are one of the most costly aspects of treatments of diabetes.[15] Two trials have demonstrated reduced amputation rates and reduced recurrence of serious foot lesions as a consequence of educational and qualified foot care.[16,17]

Eyes
All diabetic patients should have an annual eye examination (indicator 6).

Diabetic eye disease is the most common cause of blindness in the UK.[18] Appropriate intervention with laser treatment will significantly reduce blindness if it is given before significant visual loss has occurred.[19] Meta-analysis of studies of screening followed by treatment of sight-threatening retinopathy shows a high level of effectiveness.[20] A large review has shown that screening has the highest sensitivity and specificity when carried out by retinal photography or by trained and accredited optometrists.[21] New recommendations from the National Screening Committee suggest that the preferred modality is digital imaging. The sensitivity of GPs using opthalmoscopy is poor, ranging from 33% for any retinopathy to 67% for sight-threatening retinopathy. It has been estimated that comprehensive screening and treatment for diabetic retinopathy could prevent 260 new cases of blindness every year.

Lipids
All diabetic patients should have their lipid profiles measured, including total serum cholesterol, HDL, LDL and triglycerides (indicators 7 and 8). Diabetic patients with raised lipids and established ischaemic heart disease should be given lipid lowering medication. Subgroup analysis of large randomised controlled trials has identified the benefits to diabetics of lipid-lowering medication.[22,23] Most published trials on lipid lowering include comparatively small numbers of diabetics. However, compared with the non-diabetics in the studies the risk reduction for diabetics was greater. Evidence for the benefit of primary prevention of hyperlipidaemia is only available from studies with small numbers and studies in secondary or tertiary care.[24,25]

Proteinuria
Diabetic patients with proteinuria should receive treatment with ACE inhibitors (indicator 9). Elevated urinary protein excretion is a marker for increased cardiovascular morbidity and mortality. However, the cardiovascular benefits of

reducing proteinuria by interventions remains unknown.[26] Renal function declines progressively in patients who have diabetic nephropathy and that decline can be slowed by antihypertensive medication. There seems to be a beneficial effect from ACE inhibitors that is independent of the blood pressure lowering effect. This benefit has been shown in a randomised controlled trial on insulin-dependent diabetics with proteinuria ($\geq$500 mg/day).[27]

Microalbuminuria

The evidence for treatment of microalbuminuria is clear in so far as ACE inhibitors can arrest or reduce the albumin excretion rate in microalbuminuric normotensive diabetics.[28] However, a direct link with postponement of end stage renal failure has not been demonstrated.

Incipient nephropathy refers to the presence of low but abnormal levels of albumin in the urine (>30 mg/day). Without specific interventions about 80% of type 1 patients will progress to overt nephropathy over a period of 10–15 years. Again without specific interventions end stage renal disease develops in 50% of those with type 1 with overt nephropathy within 10 years and in >75% within 20 years. Treatment with ACE inhibitors is a specific intervention at all stages and the theory is therefore that treating normotensive microalbuminuric patients will postpone or prevent end stage renal disease, although this has not been proven.

The figures are different for type 2 diabetes. Without specific interventions 20–40% of type 2 patients with microalbuminuria progress to overt nephropathy, but by 20 years after onset of overt nephropathy only about 20% will have progressed to end stage renal disease.[29] It is therefore difficult to predict in this group which patients progress to end stage renal disease from the stage of microalbuminuria.

Aspirin

Diabetic patients over the age of 30 and at high risk of cardiovascular disease should probably be prescribed aspirin, as should any diabetic patient with established cardiovascular disease, unless there are specific contraindications. High-risk patients include smokers and those with a family history of coronary heart disease, as well as those suffering from hypertension, obesity, albuminuria and elevated lipid levels.

For the primary prevention of cardiovascular disease, studies have demonstrated that the daily use of aspirin reduces the risk of myocardial infarction in both type 1 and type 2 diabetics.[30,31] For the secondary prevention of cardiovascular disease, the evidence for the benefit of aspirin in diabetic patients is stronger.[32]

Monitoring

Type 1 diabetic patients should self-monitor their glucose control. This is associated with improved glycaemic control in type 1 diabetics[33] but is of uncertain value for type 2.[34]

Immunisation

All diabetic patients should receive influenza and pneumococcal vaccines (indicator 11). While there have been no direct randomised controlled trials of the benefits of these vaccines specifically for those with diabetes, the trials that have been carried out are on population groups that include diabetics, and the benefits of vaccination are clearly established for at-risk groups. A study of available evidence from case control studies and indirect cohort analysis is clearly in favour of immunisation for diabetic patients.[35]

Follow-up

Experts recommend that patients should be seen annually by a trained member of a primary health care team (indicator 10), although there is no experimental evidence to determine the best follow-up interval.

Recommended quality indicators for diabetes mellitus

Diagnosis
1 The diagnosis of diabetes should be clearly identifiable on the electronic or paper records of all known diabetics

Treatment
2 If the HbA1c level of a diabetic patient is measured as >8%, the following options should be offered: change in dietary or drug management; or explanation for raised test; or written record that higher target level is acceptable
3 HbA1c levels should be checked in diabetic patients at least every 12 months
4.1 If a diabetic has a sustained blood pressure recorded as >140/85 mmHg on 3 or more consecutive occasions then a change in non-drug or drug management should be offered
4.2 Diabetic patients with a blood pressure of >140/85 should have their blood pressure remeasured within 3 months
5.1 Diabetics should have their feet examined at least once every 12 months
5.2 If there is evidence of foot deformities, history of foot ulceration, significant vascular or neuropathic disease, the patient should be referred to an appropriate service, if not already under their care
6 All diabetic patients should have an annual fundal examination
7 All diabetic patients should have the following measurements taken for lipid profile within the last 3 years:
   a. total serum cholesterol
   b. triglycerides
8 Diabetic patients with established ischaemic heart disease and a raised fasting cholesterol (≥5 mmol/L) should be advised about dietary modification, or to take lipid-lowering medication
9 Diabetic patients with sustained proteinuria should be currently prescribed treatment with ACE inhibitors, unless contraindicated

Follow-up
10 Patients should be seen by an appropriate health care professional (GP, practice nurse, diabetic Doctor) annually
11 All diabetic patients should be offered:
   a. influenza vaccination annually
   b. pneumococcal vaccination
   unless contraindicated or intolerant

Overview of data sources used in this review

This review is based on a Medline search using the key words Diabetes Mellitus (exploded), plus clinical trial/meta-analysis/evaluation/family practice. Bibliographies of electronically extracted references were hand searched for references to further studies. In addition, the following data sources were accessed: Cochrane Library http://www.update-software.com/clibhome/clib.htm; the NHS Centre for Reviews and Dissemination http://www.york.ac.uk/inst/crd/welcome.htm; the NHS Wisdom site http://www.shef.ac.uk/uni/projects/wrp/; the NHS Electronic Library http:// www.nelh.nhs.uk/screening/diabetic-retinopathy; Bandolier http://www.jr2.ox.ac.uk/Bandolier/; the NHS HTA programme http://www.soton.ac.uk/~hta/; the BMJ site http://www.bmj.com/ for specialised area in diabetes and the biannual BMJ publication *Clinical Evidence.*

Ideally studies would be on primary care populations of diabetic patients but this was rarely the case. The review relates to all ages and types of diabetic patients in primary care. However children and pregnant women with diabetes have special needs and their care is best given through specialist hospital clinics.

References

1. Calman K. On the state of the public health. The annual report of the Chief Medical Officer of the Department of Health for the year 1997. London: The Stationery Office, 1998
2. British Diabetes Association statement. January 2000
3. Harris MI, Klein RE, Welborn TA, Knuiman MW. Onset of NIDDM occurs at least 4–7 years before clinical diagnosis. Diabetes Care 1992; 15: 815–819
4. Peters AL, Davidson MB, Schriger DL, Hasselblad. A clinical approach for the diagnosis of diabetes mellitus: an analysis using glycosylated haemoglobin levels. Journal of the American Medical Association 1996; 276: 1246–1252
5. Griffin S, Kinmonth AL. Diabetes care: the effectiveness of systems for routine surveillance for people with diabetes. The Cochrane Database of Systematic Reviews. The Cochrane Library. Last update November 1997
6. Brown SA. Studies of educational interventions and outcomes in diabetic adults: a meta-analysis revisited. Patient Education and Counseling 1990; 16(3): 189–215
7. DCCT Research Group. The effects of intensive treatment on the development and progression of long-term complications in insulin-dependent diabetes mellitus. New England Journal of Medicine 1993; 329: 977–86
8. UKPDS group 34. Effect of intensive blood-glucose control with Metformin on complications in overweight patients with type 2 diabetes. Lancet 1998; 352: 854–865
9. Butler C, Peters J, Stott N. Glycated haemoglobin and metabolic control of diabetes mellitus: external versus locally established clinical targets for primary care. British Medical Journal 1995; 310: 784–788
10. Fuller J, Stevens LK, Chaturvedi N, Holloway JF. Antihypertensive therapy in diabetes mellitus. The Cochrane Database of Systematic Reviews. The Cochrane Library. Last update August 1997
11. UKPDS group 38. Tight blood pressure control and risk of microvascular complications in type 2 diabetes. British Medical Journal 1998; 317: 703–713
12. The Heart Outcomes Prevention Evaluation Study Investigators. Effects of ramipril on cardiovascular and microvascular outcomes in people with diabetes mellitus: results of the HOPE study and MICRO-HOPE substudy. Lancet 2000; 355:
13. Boulton A, Connor H, Cavanagh P. The foot in diabetes. Chichester: Wiley, 1995
14. Apelqvist J, Larsson J, Agardh CD. Long term prognosis for diabetic patients with foot ulcers. Journal of Internal Medicine 1993; 233: 485–491
15. Lanig P, Cogley D, Klenerman L. Economic aspects of the diabetic foot. The Foot 1991; 1: 111–112
16. McCabe C, Stevenson R, Dolan A. Evaluation of a diabetic foot screening and protection programme. Diabetic Medicine 1998; 15: 80–84

17. Litzelman D, Slemenda C, Langefield C et al. Reduction of lower extremity clinical abnormalities in patients with non insulin dependant diabetes. Annals of Internal Medicine 1993; 119: 36–41

18. Evans J, Rooney C, Ashwood F, Dattani N, Wormald R. Blindness and partial sight in England and Wales: April 1990– March1991. Health Trends 1996; 28: 5–12

19. Diabetic Retinopathy Study Research Group. Photocoagulation treatment of diabetic retinopathy. Clinical applications of DRS findings. Ophthalmology 1998; 116: 297–303

20. Bachmann MO, Nelson SJ. Impact of diabetic retinopathy screening on a British district population: case detection and blindness prevention in an evidence based model. Journal of Epidemiology and Community Health 1998; 52: 45–52

21. NHS Centre for Reviews and Dissemination. Complications of diabetes: Screening for retinopathy. Effective Health Care 1999; 5(4): 1–6

22. The Long term Intervention with Pravastatin in Ischaemic Disease (LIPID) Study Program. Prevention of cardiovascular events and death with pravastatin in patients with coronary heart disease and a broad range of initial cholesterol levels. New England Journal of Medicine 1998; 339: 1349–1357

23. Pyorala K, Pedersen TR, Kjekshus J et al. Cholesterol lowering with simvastatin improves prognosis of diabetic patients with coronary heart disease. A subgroup analysis of the Scandinavian Simvastatin Survival Study (4S). Diabetes Care 1998; 20(4): 614–620

24. Downs JR, Clearfield M, Weiss et al. Primary prevention of acute coronary events with lovastatin in men and women with average cholesterol levels: results of AFCAPS/TexCAPS, Air Force/Texas Coronary Atherosclerosis Prevention Study. Journal of the American Medical Association 1998; 279(20): 1615–1622

25. Elkeles RS, Diamond JR, Poulter C et al. Cardiovascular outcomes in type 2 diabetics. A double blind placebo-controlled study of bezafibrate: the St. Mary's Ealing, Northwick Park Diabetes Cardiovascular Disease Prevention (SENDCAP) Study. Diabetes Care 1998; 21(4): 641–648

26. Sigal RJ. Cardiovascular disease in diabetes. Clinical Evidence 1999; 2: 225

27. Lewis EJ, Hunsicker LG, Bain RP, Rohde RD. The effect of angiotensin-converting enzyme inhibition on diabetic nephropathy. The Collaborative Study Group. New England Journal of Medicine 1993; 329: 1456–1462

28. Lovell HG. Are angiotensin converting enzyme inhibitors useful for normotensive diabetic patients with microalbuminuria? The Cochrane Database of Systematic Reviews. The Cochrane Library. Last update September 1997

29. American Diabetes Association: Clinical Practice Recommendations 2000. Diabetic Nephropathy. Diabetes Care 2000; 23(1):

30. Steering Committee of the Physicians' Health Study Research Group. Final report on the aspirin component of the ongoing Physicians' Health Study. New England Journal of Medicine 1989; 321(3): 129–135

31. ETDRS investigators. Aspirin effect on mortality and morbidity in patients with diabetes mellitus. Journal of the American Medical Association 1992; 268: 1292–1300

32. Antiplatelet Triallists Collaboration. Collaborative overview of randomised trials of antiplatelet therapy-1: Prevention of death, myocardial infarction and stroke by prolonged antiplatelet therapy in various categories of patients. British Medical Journal 1994; 308: 81–106

33. Evans JM, Newton RW, Ruta DA et al. Frequency of blood glucose monitoring in relation to glycaemic control: observational study with diabetes database. British Medical Journal 1999; 319: 83–86

34. Faas A, Schellevis FG, Van Eijk JT. The efficacy of self monitoring of blood glucose in NIDDM subjects: a criteria-based literature review. Diabetes Care 1997; 20(9): 1482–1486

35. Smith SA, Poland GA. Use of influenza and pneumococcal vaccines in people with diabetes. Technical review. Diabetes Care. 2000; 23(1): 95

►7

Hypertension

Tom Fahey

Importance

Since the description by Pickering that blood pressure levels in populations follows a normal distribution,[1] the science of epidemiology has sought to describe, quantify and treat those individuals with hypertension in whom the benefits of treatment outweigh the risks.[2] The advent of the randomised controlled trial in the management of hypertension now means that unbiased estimates of treatment efficacy are possible. It is now feasible to quantify the benefits and risks of managing hypertension in individuals: results from observational studies and randomised controlled trials give clear evidence on which to base clinical practice.[3,4] Finally, hypertension, because of its widespread prevalence, is managed primarily in the community by general practitioners and the primary health care team.[5]

Blood pressure follows a normal distribution in populations. Hypertension is therefore a quantitative deviation from the norm rather than a specific disease entity.[6] Blood pressure cut-off points used to define the presence of hypertension and normotension are purely arbitrary and such classification is used to establish prognosis and facilitate therapeutic decision making.[7] The disadvantage of this method of classification is twofold. First, blood pressure reading alone is one of several factors that determine cardiovascular risk and may not necessarily accurately reflect absolute risk.[7] Second, as observational studies have demonstrated, cardiovascular mortality and morbidity increases throughout the blood pressure range and most individuals lie within what would usually be considered the normal range. Therefore most of the population excess risk can be attributed to individuals with blood pressure readings in the normotensive or mild hypertension range.[6,7]

The results of observational studies on the relationship between blood pressure and the incidence of stroke and coronary heart disease can be summarised as follows:[3,7–9]

► Blood pressure has a positive, continuous and independent association with the risk of developing stroke and coronary heart disease (CHD). A prolonged reduction of 5 mmHg in usual diastolic blood pressure is associated with avoidance of at least one-third of the risk of stroke and at least one-fifth of the risk of coronary heart disease.

► No 'threshold' or 'J-shaped' relationship exists between blood pressure and subsequent risk. Thus for the majority of individuals, whether conventionally 'normotensive' or 'hypertensive', a lower blood pressure confers a lower relative risk of vascular disease. Indeed, the burden of events takes place among those individuals who are conventionally described as normotensive.

▶ Among individuals, the absolute benefits of a lower blood pressure are greatest in those who, as a consequence of their medical history or age, are at greatest risk of vascular disease.

Systematic reviews of randomised controlled trials of antihypertensive treatment have confirmed that the effect of lowering blood pressure on reduction of stroke (fatal and non-fatal) is 38%, while the reduction of CHD (fatal coronary heart disease and non-fatal myocardial infarction) is 18%. Both these results were highly statistically significant.[4,10,11]

Furthermore, the recent trials of statins[12-15] and aspirin[16,17] for the prevention of CHD are important steps forward in the evidence concerning management of hypertension. A significant proportion of hypertensive patients will benefit from aspirin and statin treatment, even if these treatments are targeted only at those with a high level of CHD risk.[18,19] Formal estimation of CHD risk has been proposed as an aid to treatment decisions regarding hypertension.[20-27] This estimation ideally entails counting and weighting major cardiovascular risk factors in addition to blood pressure itself.[28]

As a proportion of total mortality, stroke and CHD accounted for 12% and 26% of deaths in England in 1991.[29] Thus proper detection and control of hypertension in the community could have a major impact on cardiovascular morbidity and mortality in the UK.

There is some evidence that current management of hypertension leaves patients at an unacceptably high risk of cardiovascular complications and death, particularly from CHD but also from stroke.[30-35] In part this is a consequence of suboptimal blood pressure control,[36] but other factors are also important. In a recent study, the persistent excess of CHD events in treated hypertensive subjects was predicted by three factors; (1) evidence of target organ damage before treatment; (2) a history of cigarette smoking before treatment; and (3) the serum cholesterol values before and during treatment.[35] These observations support the concept that effective management of hypertension requires the identification of those at highest cardiovascular risk and the adoption of multifactorial intervention, targeting not only blood pressure levels, but also associated cardiovascular risk factors. The recent British Hypertension Society (BHS) guidelines embrace this concept and provide detailed guidance on the management of hypertension and associated cardiovascular risk factors.[37]

Review of evidence relating to indicator set

Screening

All adults should have their blood pressure measured routinely at least every 5 years until the age of 80 years (indicator 1.1). Those with high-normal values (135–139/85–89 mmHg) and those who have had high readings at any time previously should have blood pressure remeasured within 3 months (indicator 1.2).[37] The BHS recommendations for measuring blood pressure are now available on CD-ROM and should be followed.[37] Seated blood pressure recordings are generally sufficient, but standing blood pressure should be measured in elderly or diabetic patients to exclude orthostatic hypotension.

Diagnosis

Initial evaluation of hypertensive patient

It is recommended that all hypertensive patients should have a thorough history and physical examination and that repeated readings (at least 3 separate occasions) should be taken to confirm sustained high blood pressure (indicator 2). Only a limited number of routine investigations are needed. The aims are to elicit and document (indicators 4 and 5):

▶ causes of hypertension, e.g. renal disease, endocrine causes

▶ contributory factors, e.g. obesity, salt intake, excess alcohol intake

▶ complications of hypertension, e.g. previous stroke, left ventricular hypertrophy

▶ cardiovascular risk factors, e.g. smoking, family history

▶ contraindications to specific drugs, e.g. asthma (beta-blockers), gout (thiazides).

Routine investigation should be limited to:

▶ urine strip test for protein and blood

▶ serum creatinine and electrolytes

▶ blood glucose

▶ serum total: HDL cholesterol

▶ ECG.

Formal estimation of 10-year cardiovascular risk by use of the CHD chart issued by the Joint British Societies in their recommendations for the prevention of CHD is also advisable, so that baseline absolute cardiovascular risk can be established. This is a relatively new recommendation and since it is not yet widespread practice, it was not included as a quality indicator by the expert panels.

Treatment

Treatment thresholds

Drug therapy should be started in all patients with sustained systolic blood pressures ≥160 mmHg or sustained diastolic blood pressures ≥100 mmHg despite non-pharmacological measures (indicator 6).

Drug treatment is also indicated in patients with sustained systolic blood pressures of 140–159 mmHg or diastolic blood pressures of 90–99 mmHg if target organ damage is present, or there is evidence of established cardiovascular disease, or diabetes, or the 10-year CHD risk is raised (indicator 7).

A difficulty concerns the treatment decision for patients with 'mild' hypertension, averaging 140–159/90–99 mmHg, who are at variable risk depending on other risk factors. Advice to treat, or to leave untreated and observe, is based on the presence of additional cardiovascular risk factors including age, male sex, smoking, serum lipids and family history. Intuitive estimates of absolute risk are very inaccurate.[38-40] Risk estimation is improved when additional risk factors are simply counted,[41] but is significantly more accurate when all major risk factors are counted and *weighted* using risk functions derived from epidemiological studies, most commonly the Framingham risk function. The Joint British Societies recently issued recommendations on preventing CHD and included a computer programme; the Cardiac Risk Assessor and a CHD risk chart, both of which are based on the Framingham risk function,[37] recommend the use of either of these methods to estimate 10-year CHD risk and thereby help to rationalise treatment decisions for people with hypertension. A recently performed randomised controlled trial has demonstrated that use of risk charts has a significant benefit on systolic blood pressure control.[42]

Non-pharmacological treatment

Recent controlled trials have confirmed that changes in diet and lifestyle do lower blood pressure and may also reduce cardiovascular risk.[37,43] Clear verbal and written advice on the measures below should be provided for all hypertensive patients and also for those with high-normal blood pressure or a strong family history. They may lower blood pressure as much as drug monotherapy, reduce the need for drug therapy, enhance the antihypertensive effect of drugs, reduce the need for multiple drug regimens, and favourably influence overall cardiovascular risk. Conversely, failure to adopt these measures may attenuate the response to antihypertensive drugs.[37,43] Measures that lower blood pressure (indicator 8) are:

▶ weight reduction

▶ reduced salt intake

▶ limitation of alcohol consumption

▶ physical exercise

▶ increased fruit and vegetable consumption

▶ reduced total fat and saturated fat intake.

Measures to reduce cardiovascular risk:

▶ stop smoking

▶ replace saturated fat with polyunsaturated and monounsaturated fats; increase oily fish consumption; reduce total fat intake.

Pharmacological treatment

The BHS guidelines recommend that when no special indications or contraindications exist, the least expensive drug with the most supportive trial evidence, a low-dose thiazide diuretic, should be preferred. They recommend that the choice of antihypertensive should be selected against the following criteria:[37]

▶ Use a low dose of thiazide as first-line treatment unless there is a contraindication or a compelling indication for another drug class.

▶ Long-acting dihydropyridine calcium antagonists are a suitable alternative for isolated systolic hypertension in elderly patients when low-dose thiazide is not tolerated or contraindicated.

▶ Choice of drug will depend on relative indications and contraindications in individual patients (see Table 5 of BHS guidelines; indicators 9, 10).[37]

▶ Less than half of all hypertensives will be controlled on monotherapy and one-third will require 3 or more drugs.

Elderly patients

Hypertensive people over the age of 60 years deserve special consideration for several reasons. Systolic blood pressure rises steadily with increasing age, and the prevalence of hypertension including isolated systolic hypertension ($\geq$160/<90 mmHg) is more than 50% in those aged over 60 years.[44] These people have a high risk of cardiovascular complications when compared to younger hypertensives, and antihypertensive treatment of diastolic and isolated systolic hypertension reduces this risk.[10] Recent evidence also shows that antihypertensive therapy reduces the incidence of heart failure by 50%.[45]

Diabetic patients

The BHS guidelines make the following recommendations for the control of hypertension in diabetic patients:[37]

Type I diabetes

▶ Threshold for starting antihypertensive treatment is $\geq$140/90 mmHg.

▶ Target blood pressure <140/80 mmHg or lower if proteinuria is present.

▶ BP reduction and ACE inhibitors reduce the rate of decline in renal function.

Type II diabetes

▶ Threshold for starting antihypertensive treatment is $\geq$140/90 mmHg.

▶ Target blood pressure <140/80 mmHg.

▶ Optimal first-line therapy is not yet established but trial evidence supports the use of ACE inhibitors, beta-blockers, dihydropyridine calcium channel blockers, alpha-blockers and low-dose thiazide diuretics.

Patients at high absolute risk of a cardiovascular event

In the last 4 years the results of several controlled outcome trials have shown that statin treatment for secondary and primary prevention reduces major coronary events by 30%, reduces all-cause mortality significantly and is safe, simple and well tolerated.[12–15] The current recommendations from the BHS is that statin therapy is prioritised to patients at highest cardiovascular risk:[37]

▶ *Secondary prevention*: Serum total cholesterol >5.0 mmol/L in the presence of any of the following: myocardial infarction; angina; coronary artery bypass grafts (CABG) or angioplasty; non-haemorrhagic cerebrovascular disease; peripheral vascular disease; or atherosclerotic renovascular disease.

▶ *Primary prevention*: 10-year CHD risk 30% (equivalent to 10-year CVD risk of 40%) estimated formally by the Joint British Societies cardiac risk assessor programme or risk chart.

▶ Familial hypercholesterolaemia.

Pregnancy

Meta-analysis of trials of antihypertensive drugs in pregnancy show reduction in the risk of progression to severe hypertension and fewer hospital admissions.[46] Firm evidence is not available on the optimal threshold for treatment. There is consensus that treatment is essential at ≥170/110 mmHg. A recent meta-analysis suggests that treatment of mild-to-moderate hypertension (blood pressure levels ≥140/90 mmHg) is associated with adverse effects on fetal growth, so treatment at this level of blood pressure cannot be recommended.[47]

Renal disease

In patients with chronic renal impairment, hypertension accelerates the rate of loss of renal function, and good blood pressure control is essential to retard this process. Whether ACE inhibitors have a specific renoprotective effect in non-diabetic renal failure over and above their antihypertensive action remains uncertain. Meta-analysis of all controlled trials showed a 30% reduction in incidence of end stage renal failure with ACE inhibitor.[48]

Target blood pressure

The HOT trial has provided the best evidence to date on optimal blood pressure targets during antihypertensive treatment.[17] In patients with diastolic pressures of 100–115 mmHg, the optimal blood pressure based on an on-treatment analysis for reduction of cardiovascular events was reported to be 139/83 mmHg. However, hypertensive patients were apparently little disadvantaged provided blood pressure was below 150/90 mmHg (indicator 12). Reduction of blood pressure below the optimal level caused no harm. An important practical point is that the optimal blood pressure was attained, by titrating treatment in stepped-care fashion aiming for diastolic blood pressures of ≤90 ≤85 and ≤80 mmHg. With this systematic method of treatment the final diastolic blood pressure was above 90 mmHg in only 7% of patients.

Recommended quality indicators for hypertension

Screening

1.1 All adults over the age of 25 years should have had their blood pressure measured in the last 5 years

1.2 Patients with a blood pressure of ≥160/100 should have their blood pressure remeasured within 3 months

Diagnosis

2 Blood pressure should be measured on at least 3 separate days before starting drug treatment unless blood pressure > 200/110

3 The diagnosis of hypertension should be clearly identifiable on the electronic or paper records of all known hypertensives

4 Initial history should document assessment of the following within 3 months of diagnosis
   a. personal history of peripheral vascular disease
   b. diabetes
   c. hyperlipidaemia
   d. smoking status
   e. alcohol consumption

5 Initial laboratory investigations should include the following tests within 3 months of diagnosis:
   a. urine strip test for protein
   b. serum creatinine and electrolytes
   c. blood glucose
   d. serum/total cholesterol
   e. ECG

Treatment and follow-up

6 Drug therapies should be offered to all patients with sustained (on more than 3 occasions) systolic BP >/= 160 mmHg or sustained diastolic BP >/= 100 mmHg despite up to 6 months of non-pharmacological measures, unless contraindicated or intolerant

7 Drug treatment is offered in patients with sustained (on more than 3 occasions) systolic BPs of 140–159 mmHg or diastolic BPs 90–99 mmHg if despite 6 months of non-pharmacological measures :
   a. target organ damage is present (defined as an abnormal result on any of the tests/exams that pass)
   b. there is evidence of established cardiovascular disease
   c. the patient is diabetic
   d. the 10-year CHD risk is ≥ 15%

8 All patients with a diagnosis of hypertension should have the following non-pharmacological measures recommended:
   a. weight reduction if BMI >30
   b. limitation of alcohol consumption

9 Unless clear contraindications are recorded, non-diabetic patients should currently be prescribed as first-line therapy either a thiazide diuretic or a beta-blocker

10 Patients with the conditions below should not be treated with the following drugs:
   a. Beta-blockers for patients with a history of asthma
   b. ACE inhibitors for pregnant women

11 Patients prescribed antihypertensive medication should have their blood pressure recorded at least once per year

12 Patients with sustained high readings (>150/90 on 3 or more occasions) who are already taking antihypertensive medication should be offered a change in therapy

13 Patients prescribed ACE inhibitors should have had their renal function checked :
   a. within the 6 months before starting treatment
   b. 1 month after the start of treatment

The findings of prospective observational data and the HOT trial data have to be balanced against the current control of hypertension in UK primary care. In most cross-sectional studies, only half of hypertensive patients are deemed to be controlled when the target blood pressure is ≤ 160/90.[44,49,50]

Follow-up

The frequency of follow-up for treated patients after adequate blood pressure control is attained depends upon factors such as the severity of the hypertension, variability of blood pressure, complexity of the treatment regimen, patient compliance, and the need for non-pharmacological advice.[37] The review interval should not generally exceed 6 months. Those who have been hypertensive in the past, or who have untreated mild hypertension and a low estimated 10-year CHD/CVD risk, should have their blood pressure measured and their 10-year CHD/CVD risk estimated annually (indicator 11, though CHD risk was not included in the indicator by the panels).

The routine for follow-up visits should be simple: measure blood pressure and weight; enquire about general health, side-effects and treatment problems; reinforce advice on non-pharmacological measures; and test urine for proteinuria annually. There is some evidence that patients taking ACE inhibitors with risk factors that predispose them to uraemia (old age, peripheral vascular disease, concomitant treatment with non-steroidal drugs or high-dose diuretics) do not have their blood urea, creatinine and electrolytes checked by their general practitioner (indicator 13).[51]

A formal system of recall for those who miss routine appointments, using the practice computer, is recommended by the BHS.[37] However, a recent systematic review of interventions designed to enhance detection, adherence and control of hypertension highlights the fact that there is little evidence to support most of these management strategies.[52]

Overview of data sources used in this review

The principal data source for this review was the recently published guidelines of the management of hypertension from the British Hypertension Society.[37] In addition, evidence has been sought through MEDLINE and EMBASE searches, and the Cochrane Library has been used as a source for systematic reviews and randomised controlled trials.

References

1. Swales J. Hypertension: the past, the present and the future. In: Swales J, ed. Textbook of hypertension. Oxford: Blackwell Scientific, 1994: 1–7
2. Rose GA. Hypertension in the community. In: Bulpitt CJ, ed. Epidemiology of hypertension. Amsterdam: Elsevier, 1985: 1–23
3. MacMahon S. Blood pressure and the risks of cardiovascular disease. In: Swales J, ed. Textbook of hypertension. Oxford: Blackwell Scientific, 1994: 46–57
4. Collins R, Peto R. Antihypertensive drug therapy: effects on stroke and coronary heart disease. In: Swales J, ed. Textbook of hypertension. Oxford: Blackwell Scientific, 1994: 1156–1164
5. Tudor-Hart J. Hypertension: community control of high blood pressure. Oxford: Radcliffe Medical Press, 1993

6. Whelton P, He J, Klag M. Blood pressure in westernized populations. In: Swales J, ed. Textbook of hypertension. Oxford: Blackwell Scientific, 1994; 11–21
7. Whelton P. Epidemiology of hypertension. Lancet 1994; 344: 101–106
8. Prospective stroke collaborators. Cholesterol, diastolic blood pressure, and stroke: 13 000 strokes in 450 000 people in 45 prospective cohorts. Lancet 1995; 346: 1647–1653
9. MacMahon S, Peto R, Cutler J et al. Blood pressure, stroke, and coronary heart disease. Part 1, prolonged differences in blood pressure: prospective observational studies corrected for the regression dilution bias. Lancet 1990; 335: 765–774
10. Mulrow CD, Cornell JA, Herrera CR, Kadri A, Farnett L, Aguilar C. Hypertension in the elderly: implications and generalizability of randomised trials. Journal of the American Medical Association 1994; 272: 1932–1938
11. Insua J, Sacks H, Lau T et al. Drug treatment of hypertension in the elderly: a meta-analysis. Annals of Internal Medicine 1994; 121: 355–362
12. Scandinavian Simvastatin Survival Study Group. Randomised trial of cholesterol lowering in 4444 patients with coronary heart disease: the Scandinavian Simvastatin Survival Study (4S). Lancet 1994; 344: 1383–1389
13. Shepherd J et al. Prevention of coronary heart disease with pravastatin in men with hypercholesterolemia. New England Journal of Medicine 1995; 333: 1301–1307
14. Sacks FM et al. The effect of pravastatin on coronary events after myocardial infarction in patients with average cholesterol levels. New England Journal of Medicine 1996; 335: 1001–1009
15. Downs JR et al. Primary prevention of acute coronary events with lovastatin in men and women with average cholesterol levels. Results of AFCAPS/TexCAPS. Journal of the American Medical Association 1998; 279: 1615–1622
16. The Medical Research Council's General Practice Research Framework. Thrombosis prevention trial: randomised trial of low-intensity oral anticoagulation with warfarin and low-dose aspirin in the primary prevention of ischaemic heart disease in men at increased risk. Lancet 1998; 351: 233–241
17. Hansson L et al, for the HOT Study Group. Effects of intensive blood-pressure lowering and low-dose aspirin in patients with hypertension: principal results of the Hypertension Optimal Treatment (HOT) randomised trial. Lancet 1998; 351: 1755–1762
18. Haq IU, Jackson PR, Yea WW, Ramsay LE. Implications of recent trials with lipid-lowering drugs for hypertension management. Journal of Hypertension 1996; 14: 1502
19. Hasnain S, Webster J, McLay JS. Cardiovascular risk in hypertension: implications of the Sheffield table for lipid-lowering strategy. Journal of Human Hypertension 1998; 12: 469–471
20. Jackson R. Which hypertensive patients should be treated? Lancet 1994; 343: 496–497
21. Kannel WB. Potency of vascular risk factors as the basis for antihypertensive therapy. European Heart Journal 1992; 13 (suppl G): 34–42
22. Alderman MH. Blood pressure management: individualized treatment based on absolute risk and the potential for benefit. Annals of Internal Medicine 1993; 119: 329–335
23. Davey Smith G, Egger M. Who benefits from medical interventions? Treating low risk patients can be a high risk strategy. British Medical Journal 1994; 308: 72–74
24. Menard J, Chatellier G. Mild hypertension: the mysterious viability of a faulty concept. Journal of Hypertension 1995; 13: 1071–1077
25. Jackson RT, Sackett DL. Guidelines for managing raised blood pressure. Evidence based or evidence burdened? British Medical Journal 1996; 313: 64–65
26. Ramsay LE, Wallis EJ, Yeo WW, Jackson PR. The rationale for differing national recommendations for the treatment of hypertension. American Journal of Hypertension 1998; 11: 79S–88S
27. Core Services Committee. Guidelines for the management of mildly raised blood pressure in New Zealand. Ministry of Health: Wellington, 1995
28. Joint British recommendations on prevention of coronary heart disease in clinical practice. Heart 1998; 80(suppl 2): S1–S29
29. Department of Health. The health of the nation. A strategy for health in England. London: HMSO, 1992
30. Fahey TP, Peters TJ. A general practice based study examining the absolute risk of cardiovascular disease in treated hypertensive patients. British Journal of General Practice 1996; 46: 655–670
31. Isles CG et al. Mortality in patients of the Glasgow blood pressure clinic. Journal of Hypertension 1986; 4: 141–156
32. Clausen J, Jenson G. Blood pressure and mortality: an epidemiological survey with 10 years follow-up. Journal of Human Hypertension 1992; 6: 53–59
33. Thirlmer HL, Lund-Larsen PG, Tverdal A. Is blood pressure treatment as effective in a population setting as in controlled trials? Results from a prospective study. Journal of Hypertension 1994; 12: 481–490

34. Merlo J et al. Incidence of myocardial infarction in elderly men being treated with antihypertensive drugs: population based cohort study. British Medical Journal 1996; 313: 457–461

35. Andersson OK et al. Survival in treated hypertension: follow up study after two decades. British Medical Journal 1998; 317: 167–171

36. Du X et al. Case-control study of stroke and the quality of hypertension control in north west England. British Medical Journal 1997; 314: 272–276

37. Ramsay LE, Williams B, Johnston G et al. Guidelines for the management of hypertension: report of the third working party of the British Hypertension Society. Journal of Human Hypertension 1999; 13: 569–592

38. Montgomery AA, Fahey T, Peters TJ, MacKintosh C, Sharp D. Estimation of cardiovascular risk in hypertensive patients in general practice. British Journal of General Practice 2000; 50: 127–128

39. Grover S et al. Do doctors accurately assess coronary risk in their patients? Preliminary results of the coronary health assessment study. British Medical Journal 1995; 310: 975–978

40. Evans J St BT, Harries C, Dennis I, Dean J. General practitioners' tacit and stated policies in the prescription of lipid lowering agents. British Journal of General Practice 1995; 45: 15–18

41. Grover SA, Coupal L, Hu X-P. Identifying adults at increased risk of coronary disease. How well do the current cholesterol guidelines work? Journal of the American Medical Association 1995; 274: 801–806

42. Montgomery AA,. Fahey T, Peters TJ, MacKintosh C, and Sharp D. Evaluation of a computer-based clinical decision support system and chart guidelines in the management of hypertension in primary care: a randomised controlled trial. British Medical Journal, 2000; 320: 686–690

43. Ebrahim S, Davey Smith G. Lowering blood pressure: a systematic review of sustained effects of non-pharmacological interventions. Journal of Public Health Medicine 1998; 20: 441–448

44. Colhoun HM, Dong W, Poulter NR. Blood pressure screening, management and control in England: results from the health survey for England 1994. Journal of Hypertension 1998; 16: 747–752

45. Kostis JB et al for the SHEP Cooperative Research Group. Prevention of heart failure by antihypertensive drug treatment in older persons with isolated systolic hypertension. Journal of the American Medical Association 1997; 278: 212–216

46. Collins R, Wallenburg HCS. Pharmacological prevention and treatment of hypertensive disorders in pregnancy. In: Chalmers I, Enkin M, Keirse MJNC, eds. Effective care in pregnancy and childbirth, vol. 1: 166, Pregnancy, 1992: 382–402

47. von Dadelszen P, Ornstein M, Bull S, Logan A, Magee L. Fall in mean arterial pressure and fetal growth restriction in pregnancy hypertension: a meta analysis. Lancet 2000; 355: 87–92

48. Giatras 1, Lau J, Levey AS, for the Angiotensin-Converting-Enzyme Inhibition and Progressive Renal Disease Study Group. Effect of angiotensin-converting enzyme inhibitors on the progression of nondiabetic renal disease: a meta-analysis of randomized trials. Annals of Internal Medicine 1997; 127: 337–345

49. Fahey T, Lancaster T. The detection and management of hypertension in the elderly of Northamptonshire. Journal of Public Health Medicine 1995; 17: 57–62

50. Cranney M, Barton S. Performance indicators in primary care. British Medical Journal 1999; 318: 804

51. Kalra P, Kumwenda M, MacDowall P, Roland M. Questionnaire study and audit of use of angiotensin converting enzyme inhibitor and monitoring in general practice: the need for guidelines to prevent renal failure. British Medical Journal 1999; 318: 234–237

52. Ebrahim S. Detection, adherence and control of hypertension for the prevention of stroke: a systematic review. Health Technology Assessment 1998; 2: 11

▶8

Osteoarthritis

Martin Underwood

Importance

Osteoarthritis is a common problem.[1] Increasing age is the most important predictor and demographic changes mean that it will become more common. Estimating the prevalence of osteoarthritis is difficult. Nearly everyone over the age of 65 has some changes visible on x-ray, and 60% of these will have moderate or severe changes in at least one joint.[2] In an American study of over 65-year-olds based on history, 30% of women and 17% of men had osteoarthritis and, based on examination, 41% of women and 20% of men were considered to have osteoarthritis.[3] UK data suggest that around 12% of those aged 65 or over are affected by osteoarthritis.[4] Others estimate that osteoarthritis causes pain or dysfunction in 20% of elderly people.[5] Only cardiovascular disease results in greater disability.[6]

Apart from surgery there is no treatment that slows the degenerative process. Primary care management should therefore target pain and disability.[7]

Review of evidence relating to indicator set

Screening

Although there is observational evidence that those who are obese are at higher risk of developing osteoarthritis,[8] screening is not recommended.

Diagnosis

Osteoarthritis is usually a disease of older people.[9] Patients commonly complain of:

▶ pain worsened by activity or weightbearing and relieved by rest

▶ stiffness after inactivity that is short lived and relieved by exercise.

The most frequently affected joints are:

▶ knees

▶ hips

▶ proximal and distal interphalangeal joints

▶ first carpometacarpal joints

▶ cervical and lumbar spine.

The wrists, elbows, shoulders and ankles are rarely affected.

There may be little or no joint effusion. Bony swelling, localised tenderness, secondary synovitis and joint crepitus may be present. The differential diagnosis includes:

- other joint diseases, e.g. rheumatoid arthritis, gout or pseudogout
- periarticular conditions, e.g. tendonitis, bursitis, impingement or neoplasm
- other local rheumatological problems, e.g. referred pain from the hip causing knee pain
- other generalised rheumatological disorders, e.g. polymyalgia rheumatica or fibromyalgia.

Evaluation should cover:[10,11]

- the patient's symptoms
- their impact on activities of daily living
- identification of symptoms of generalised disorders
- previous trauma
- effect of previous treatments
- use of self-medication including over-the-counter drugs and complementary therapies.

Joint examination should assess pain, bony swelling, range of movement and effusion.

Laboratory tests
Laboratory investigations are not usually required.[9]

Radiography
X-ray changes of osteoarthritis are common but only 60% of these are associated with symptoms.[5,12,13] Radiological evidence is not necessarily required for the diagnosis of osteoarthritis of the knee, hip or hand.[14–16]

The Royal College of Radiologists' (RCR) guidelines on making best use of a department of clinical radiology have made recommendations regarding hip and knee x-rays in adults (Table 8.1).[17] These rely on expert opinion and have the endorsement of respected authorities.

Treatment
Drugs form only one part of the management of osteoarthritis. The importance of non-pharmacological techniques should be emphasised.[11]

Pharmacological therapies

Analgesics
There is little evidence comparing paracetamol and paracetamol/mild opiate

Table 8.1 RCR guidelines[17]

Clinical problem	Investigation	Recommendation	Comment
Hip pain: full movement	X-ray pelvis	Not routinely indicated	X-ray only if symptoms and signs persist or complex history (e.g. possible avascular necrosis)
Hip pain: limited movement	X-ray pelvis	Not indicated initially	Symptoms often transient X-ray if hip replacement is considered
Knee pain: without locking or restriction in movement	X-ray knee	Not routinely indicated	Symptoms frequently arise from soft tissues and these will not be demonstrated on x-ray Osteoarthritis changes common X-rays needed when considering surgery
Knee pain: with locking, restricted movement or effusion (? loose body)	X-ray knee	Indicated	To identify radio-opaque loose bodies

combinations with placebo for the treatment of osteoarthritis. They are widely used, however, and have a good side-effect profile. Two trials suggest that paracetamol is as effective as non-steroidal anti-inflammatory drugs (NSAIDs) for treatment of osteoarthritis of the knee.[18] A trial of paracetamol versus paracetamol plus codeine failed to show an additional benefit from codeine for hip osteoarthritis.[19] For those patients with osteoarthritis who wish to take medication, paracetamol is an appropriate first-line medication[20] (indicator 1).

Non-steroidal anti-inflammatory drugs

NSAIDs are widely used for pain by those with osteoarthritis, but their use is associated with risks such as the development of gastrointestinal side-effects, renal insufficiency, hepatic toxicity, sodium retention and loss of hypertension control.[21] Risk factors for gastrointestinal bleeding include: age over 65; past history of peptic ulcer disease; concomitant use of steroids and/or anticoagulants; smoking; and alcohol.[20]

Several trials have shown NSAIDs to be superior to placebo in the treatment of osteoarthritis of the knee.[18] There is probably little to choose between different NSAIDs in terms of effectiveness in the treatment of osteoarthritis of the hip[22] and knee.[23] A meta-analysis of the risk of gastrointestinal side-effects found that ibuprofen had the lowest risk, and the next safest was diclofenac. The relative risks for some other NSAIDs compared to ibuprofen were piroxicam 3.8, ketoprofen 4.2 and azopropazone 9.2[24] (indicator 2).

Prevention of gastrointestinal damage from NSAIDs

A meta-analysis of randomised controlled trials calculated the numbers needed to treat with H_2 antagonists or misoprostol to prevent peptic ulceration identified on gastroscopy at different levels of risk (Table 8.2). They recommend that only high-risk patients receive H_2 antagonist or misoprostol (indicator 3). The risk is highest earlier on in treatment, suggesting that if used they should be administered as soon as possible.[25] The possible side-effects of H_2 antagonist and misoprostol were not considered.

Table 8.2 Number needed to treat to prevent one NSAID-induced ulcer NNT (95% CI)

	Gastric ulcer		Duodenal ulcer	
	Baseline risk		Baseline risk	
	3%	30%	3%	30%
H_2 antagonist Short term <2/52	Not significant	Not significant	Insufficient data	Insufficient data
H_2 antagonist Long term >4/52	Not significant	Not significant	54 (41–136)	6 (4–18)
Misoprostol Short term <2/52	35 (34–39)	4 (3–4)	36 (34–60)	4 (3–7)
Misoprostol Long term >4/52	47 (41–58)	5 (5–7)	47 (40–65)	8 (4–8)

A Cochrane review of prevention of NSAID-induced gastrointestinal problems[26] found that:

1. Misoprostol reduced the risk of endoscopic ulcers and that a dose of 800 µg/day (relative risk [RR] 0.18) was more effective than 400 µg/day (RR 0.38) at reducing gastric ulcers. A dose response was not found for gastric ulcers.

2. Standard doses of H_2 antagonists are effective at reducing the risk of duodenal ulcers (RR 0.36 at 3 months) but not gastric ulcers.

3. Double doses of both H_2 antagonists and proton pump inhibitors reduced the risk of developing duodenal (RR 0.26 and RR 0.19 respectively) and gastric ulcers (RR 0.44 and RR 0.37 respectively) and were better tolerated than misoprostol.

Only one trial (of patients with rheumatoid arthritis) used clinically important complications as an outcome.[27] Misoprostol 800 µg/day reduced the risk of complications over a 6-month period from 0.95% to 0.57%; 17% of those on misoprostol and 9% of those on placebo had diarrhoea or abdominal pain (indicator 3). A non-systematic review identified four studies that suggested that the coprescription of misoprostol with NSAIDs is cost-effective, at least for high-risk patients, and two studies that suggested that it was not.[28]

A number of selective Cox-2 inhibitors that have much less effect on the gastric mucosa have been, or are about to be, marketed[29]. It has been suggested that clinical outcome and endoscopic studies of Cox-2 inhibitors mean that NSAID use and prophylaxis might need reconsidering[26]. Other effects on the gastrointestinal and other systems mean that caution is still needed in case there are unexpected late risks from Cox-2 use.[30]

An Australian quasi-experimental study of advice and information to practitioners led to a 28% decrease in NSAID deliveries to pharmacies and a 70% reduction in admissions for gastrointestinal disorders over a 5-year period in the intervention district compared to a comparison district (indicator 1).[31]

Topical NSAIDs

A meta-analysis of 12 studies of chronic conditions (osteoarthritis, tendinitis) found the pooled relative benefit of topical NSAIDs, when compared to placebo, to be 2 (95% CI 1.5–2.7) with an NNT of 3.1 (95% CI 2.7–3.8).[32] Topical NSAIDs may have fewer side-effects than oral NSAIDs but patients may still suffer systemic side-effects.

Capsaicin

Meta-analysis of three trials of capsaicin for osteoarthritis supported its usefulness. The odds ratio for an improvement with capsaicin was 4.36 (95% CI 2.77–6.88). It should be noted that it was not possible to fully blind participants because of the irritant effects of capsaicin.[33]

Rubefacients

No placebo-controlled trials of rubefacients were identified.

Glucosamine and chondroitin

The nutraceuticals chondroitin and glucosamine are used for treatment of osteoarthritis. Chondroitin is a glycosaminoglycan and glucosamine is required for the synthesis of glycosaminoglycans.[34] A systematic review of 15 placebo-controlled trials found evidence of moderate (glucosamine) or large (chondroitin) effects on pain.[35] Publication bias and quality issues suggest that these effects may be exaggerated.

Non-pharmacological therapies

Exercise

A systematic review identified 11 trials of exercise therapy for osteoarthritis of the hip or knee.[36] Results suggest that exercise therapy has a small to moderate beneficial effect on pain, small beneficial effects on self-reported and observed disability and moderate to great beneficial effects according to patients' global assessment of effect.

Yoga

There is some evidence from two small studies to suggest that yoga and hand exercises might help osteoarthritis of the hand.[37]

Ultrasound

A meta-analysis of ultrasound for musculoskeletal disorders pooled results from 13 trials of ultrasound including a sham-ultrasound control. A number of different conditions were included, including knee osteoarthritis. There was no significant difference between the two groups. The authors concluded that any therapeutic effect of ultrasound was insignificant compared to the effects of NSAIDs.[38] The fact that trials on a number of conditions were pooled means that these results do not necessarily exclude an effect in individual conditions.

Laser

A Cochrane review[39] identified five trials of laser therapy for osteoarthritis. The results showed no clear evidence of benefit.

Acupuncture

Ernst[40] identified 13 trials of acupuncture for osteoarthritis. Seven reported positive results and 6 did not. Most of the positive trials had serious methodological flaws. The two double-blind randomised controlled trials concluded that acupuncture was not superior to sham needling. One subsequent study does suggest a benefit from acupuncture for knee osteoarthritis.[41]

Homoeopathy

A meta-analysis of placebo controlled trials of homeopathy did not identify any studies of osteoarthritis.[42]

Transcutaneous electrical nerve stimulation (TENS)

Puett & Griffin[7] identified three studies of TENS. The active and treatment groups both showed an overall improvement. All three studies reported superior pain control in the active group.

Pulsed electromagnetic fields

Puett & Griffin[7] identified one study using pulsed electromagnetic fields to treat osteoarthritis of the knee. This small trial found some reduction in pain and improvement in overall patient assessment.

Spa therapy

Ernst & Pittler[43] identified three randomised controlled trials of spa therapy; one was on patients with osteoarthritis and indicated some benefit. They concluded that the evidence was insufficient to prove or disprove a benefit from spa therapy.

Hydrotherapy

A Cochrane review[44] identified two small trials of hydrotherapy for osteoarthritis of the hip. One showed benefit and one did not show benefit compared to usual care.

Assistive devices

The use of a walking stick, splint or appropriate footwear is thought to improve quality of life and reduce the risk of falling.[9]

Knee taping

A single study of taping the patella for patients with osteoarthritis of the knee found a 25% reduction in knee pain with medial taping.[45]

Other physical treatments
Other physical treatments that have been used include heat treatment and cold treatment. There are few objective data to support their use.

Educational interventions
Superio-Cabuslay et al.[46] identified 10 educational intervention studies of patients with osteoarthritis. These did not show a statistically significant improvement in pain or functional disability.

Weight loss
Obesity is a major risk factor for the development of knee osteoarthritis. The odds of those with a body mass index in the highest third of the population developing osteoarthritis of the knee are 18.3 higher than for those in the lowest third.[7] Observational data suggest that for obese women each 11 pounds of weight loss reduces the risk of developing knee osteoarthritis by around 50%.[47]

Three small intervention studies of weight loss as a treatment for osteoarthritis were identified. Two used appetite-suppressant drugs and one used powdered meal replacements. One found that weight loss was associated with improved mobility, one found no effect and the third found an improvement in a composite measure of weight loss and mobility.[48-50] A review of trials of weight reduction for patients with hypertension, some using quite intense interventions, found that modest weight loss (in the order of 3–9%) could be achieved.[51]

Invasive therapies

Intra-articular steroid injections
There is some evidence from a small number of randomised controlled trials that intra-articular corticosteroids have a significant short-term benefit (1–3 weeks) for knee osteoarthritis.[52,53] Frequent injections may cause damage to weightbearing joints.[20]

Arthroscopic lavage
Arthroscopic lavage may be useful for some patients with osteoarthritis of the knee.[20] One randomised controlled trial has shown a benefit.[53] Its role in the management of osteoarthritis is not yet clear.

Surgery
Numerous studies have shown knee and hip joint replacements to be effective.[55,56] Mortality is low, in the order of 0.34–0.4%.[57,58] A number of consensus statements have concluded that the principal indications for hip replacement are pain and functional limitation.[59] Best results are obtained in those aged 45–75 years, who are fitter preoperatively, without concurrent illnesses, who are better educated and who have good social support[60] (indicator 4).

Follow-up

There are no recommendations for the follow-up of patients with osteoarthritis except for those treated with NSAIDs. Patients with renal, cardiac or hepatic impairment who are prescribed NSAIDs should have their renal function monitored.[21]

Recommended quality indicators for osteoarthritis

Treatment
1 Patients with a new diagnosis of osteoarthritis who wish to take medication for joint symptoms should be offered a trial of paracetamol if not already tried
2 If NSAIDs are considered, ibuprofen should be considered for first-line treatment unless contraindicated or intolerant
3 Patients with osteoarthritis prescribed oral NSAIDs who are at high risk of gastrointestinal side-effects (past history of dyspepsia or known peptic ulcer) should be considered for a coprescription of PPIs, H_2 antagonists or misoprostol, unless contraindicated or intolerant
4 Patients with severe symptomatic osteoarthritis of the knee or hip who have failed to respond to conservative therapy should be offered referral to an orthopaedic surgeon for consideration of joint replacement

---

Overview of data sources used in this review

The Cochrane database and the DARE database were searched for completed non-systematic and systematic reviews. Other primary research and review articles in areas not covered by the previously identified systematic reviews were identified from Medline.

Further reading

The most useful further reading are the various Cochrane reviews on the subject of osteoarthritis. Two consensus statements on the management of osteoarthritis are also helpful.

Anonymous. Guidelines for the diagnosis, investigation and management of osteoarthritis of the hip and knee. Report of a Joint Working Group of the British Society for Rheumatology and the Research Unit of the Royal College of Physicians. Journal of the Royal College of Physicians of London 1993; 27(4): 391–396

Dickson J, Brett M, Clark J, Hosie G, Maskrey N, Rodley R. Partnership in practice. The management of osteoarthritis. PCR Northallerton, 1996

References

1. Gabriel SE. Update on the epidemiology of the rheumatic diseases. Current Opinion in Rheumatology 1996; 8(2): 96–100
2. Croft P. Review of UK data on the rheumatic diseases – 3 Osteoarthritis. British Journal of Rheumatology 1990; 29(5): 391–395
3. Mikkelsen WM, Dodge HJ, Duff IF et al. Estimates of the prevalence of rheumatic diseases in the population of Tecumseh, Michigan, 1959–1960. Journal of Chronic Diseases 1967; 20(6): 351–369

4. Dieppe P, Kirwan J. The localisation of osteoarthritis. British Journal of Rheumatology 1994; 33(3): 201–203

5. Lawrence JS, Brenuner JM, Bier F. Osteo-arthrosis. Prevalence in the population and relationship between symptoms and x-ray changes. Annals of the Rheumatic Diseases 1966; 25(1): 1–24

6. Wright V. Osteoarthritis. British Medical Journal 1989; 299(6714): 1476–1477

7. Puett DW, Griffin MR. Published trials of non-medicinal and noninvasive therapies of hip and knee osteoarthritis. Annals of Internal Medicine 1994; 121(2): 133–140

8. Cooper C, Snow S, McAlindon TE et al. Risk factors for the incidence and progression of radiographic knee osteoarthritis. Arthritis and Rheumatism 2000; 43(5): 995–1000

9. Hutton CW. Osteoarthritis. In: Weatherall DJ, Ledingham JGC, Warrell DA, eds. Oxford textbook of medicine, 3rd edn. Oxford: Oxford University Press, 1996: 2975–2983

10. Anonymous. Guidelines for the diagnosis, investigation and management of osteoarthritis of the hip and knee. Report of a Joint Working Group of the British Society for Rheumatology and the Research Unit of the Royal College of Physicians. Journal of the Royal College of Physicians of London 1993; 27(4): 391–396

11. Dickson J, Brett M, Clark J, Hosie G, Maskrey N, Rodley R. Partnership in practice. The management of osteoarthritis. PCR Northallerton, 1996

12. Claessens AA, Schouten JSAG, van den Ouweland FA, Valkenburg HA. Do clinical findings associate with radiographic osteoarthritis of the knee? Annals of the Rheumatic Diseases 1990; 49(10): 771–774

13. Davis MA, Ettinger WH, Neuhaus JM et al. Correlates of knee pain among US adults with and without radiographic knee osteoarthritis. Journal of Rheumatology 1992; 19(12): 1943–1949

14. Altman R, Asch E, Bloch D et al. Development of criteria for the classification and reporting of osteoarthritis: classification of osteoarthritis of the knee. Arthritis and Rheumatism 1986; 29(8): 1039–1049

15. Altman R, Alarcon G, Appelrouth D et al. The American College of Rheumatology criteria for the classification and reporting of osteoarthritis of the hand. Arthritis and Rheumatism 1990; 33(11): 1601–1610

16. Altman R, Alarcon G, Appelrouth D et al. The American College of Rheumatology criteria for the classification and reporting of osteoarthritis of the hip. Arthritis and Rheumatism 1991; 34(5): 505–514

17. Royal College of Radiologists. Making the best use of a department of clinical radiology. Guidelines for doctors, 4th edn. London: Royal College of Radiologists, 1998

18. Towheed TE, Hochberg MC. A systematic review of randomized controlled trials of pharmacological therapy in osteoarthritis of the knee, with an emphasis on trial methodology. Seminars in Arthritis and Rheumatism 1997; 26(5): 755–770

19. Kjaersgaard-Andersen P, Nafei A, Skov O et al. Codeine plus paracetamol versus paracetamol in longer-term treatment of chronic pain due to osteoarthritis of the hip. A randomised, double-blind, multi-centre study. Pain 1990; 43(3): 309–318

20. Lane NE, Thompson JM. Management of osteoarthritis in the primary-care setting: an evidence-based approach to treatment. American Journal of Medicine 1997; 103(6a): 25s–30s

21. Anonymous. British National Formulary 39 March 10.1.1 London: British Medical Association & Royal Pharmaceutical Society, 2000: 447–448

22. Towheed T, Shea B, Wells G, Hochberg M. Analgesia and non-aspirin, non-steroidal anti-inflammatory drugs for osteoarthritis of the hip. (Cochrane review). In: The Cochrane Library, issue 4. Oxford: Update Software, 1999

23. Watson MC, Brookes ST, Kirwan JR, Faulkner A. Non-aspirin, non-steroidal anti-inflammatory drugs for osteoarthritis of the knee (Cochrane review), In: The Cochrane Library, issue 4. Oxford: Update Software, 1999

24. Henry D, Lim LL, Garcia Rodriguez LA et al. Variability in risk of gastrointestinal complications with individual non-steroidal anti-inflammatory drugs: results of a collaborative meta-analysis. British Medical Journal 1996; 312(7046): 1563–1566

25. Koch M, Dezi A, Ferrario F, Capurso I. Prevention of nonsteroidal anti-inflammatory drug-induced gastrointestinal mucosal injury. A meta-analysis of randomized controlled clinical trials. Archives of Internal Medicine 1996; 156(20): 2321–2332

26. Rostom A, Wells G, Tugwell P, Welch V, Dube C, McGowan J, Prevention of chronic NSAID induced upper gastrointestinal toxicity (Cochrane review). In: The Cochrane Library, Issue 3. Oxford: Update Software, 2000

27. Silverstein FE, Graham DY, Senior JR et al. Misoprostol reduces serious gastrointestinal complications in patients with rheumatoid arthritis receiving nonsteroidal anti-inflammatory drugs. A randomized, double-blind, placebo-controlled trial. Annals of Internal Medicine 1995; 123(4): 241–249

28. Phillips AC, Polisson RP, Simon LS. NSAIDs and the elderly, toxicity and economic implications. Drugs and Aging 1997; 10(2): 119–130

29. Hawkey CJ. Cox-2 inhibitors. Lancet 1999; 353(9149): 307–314
30. Wollheim FA. Selective Cox-2 inhibition in man – therapeutic breakthrough or cosmetic advance. Rheumatology 2000; 39(9): 935–938
31. May FW, Rowett DS, Gilbert AJ, McNeece JI, Hurley E. Outcomes of an educational-outreach service for community medical practitioners: non-steroidal anti-inflammatory drugs. Medical Journal of Australia 1999; 170(4): 471–474
32. Moore RA, Tramer MR, Carroll D, Wiffen PJ, McQuay HJ. Quantitative systematic review of topically applied non-steroidal anti-inflammatory drugs. British Medical Journal 1998; 316(7128): 333–338
33. Zhang WY, Li Wan Po A. The effectiveness of topically applied capsaicin: a meta-analysis. European Journal of Clinical Pharmacology 1994; 46(6): 517–522
34. Towheed TE, Anastassiades TA. Glucosamine and chondroitin for treating symptoms of osteoarthritis. Journal of the American Medical Association 2000; 283(11) 1483–1484
35. McAlindon TE, LaValley MP, Gulin JP, Felson DT. Glucosamine and chondroitin for treatment of osteoarthritis. A systematic quality assessment and meta analysis. Journal of the American Medical Association 2000; 283(1): 1469–1475
36. van Baar ME, Assendelft WJJ, Dekker J, Oostendorp RAB, Bijlsma JW. Effectiveness of exercise therapy in patients with osteoarthritis of the hip or knee. Arthritis and Rheumatism 1999; 42(7): 1361–1369
37. Garfinkel M, Schumacher HR Jr. Yoga. Rheumatic Diseases Clinics of North America 2000; 26(1): 125–132
38. Gam AN, Johannsen F. Ultrasound therapy in musculoskeletal disorders: a meta-analysis. Pain 1995; 63(1): 85–91
39. Brosseau L, Welch V, Wells G et al. Low level laser therapy (classes I, II and III) for the treatment of osteoarthritis (Cochrane review). In: The Cochrane Library, issue 3. Oxford: Update Software, 2000
40. Ernst E. Acupuncture as a symptomatic treatment for osteoarthritis: a systematic review. Scandinavian Journal of Rheumatology 1997; 26(6): 444–447
41. Berman BM, Singh BB, Lao L et al. A randomized trial of acupuncture as an adjunctive therapy in osteoarthritis of the knee. Rheumatology 1999; 38(4): 346–354
42. Linde K, Clausius N, Ramirez G et al. Are the clinical effects of homeopathy placebo effects? A meta-analysis of placebo-controlled trials. Lancet 1997; 350(9081): 834–843
43. Ernst E, Pittler MH. [How effective is spa treatment? A systematic review of randomised studies] Deutsche Medizinische Wochenschrift 1998; 123(10): 273–277
44. Verhagen AP, de Vet HCW, de Bie RA, Kessels AGH, Boers M, Knipschild PG. Balneotherapy for rheumatoid arthritis and osteoarthritis (Cochrane review). In: The Cochrane Library, issue 3. Oxford: Update Software, 2000
45. Cushnaghan J, McCarthy C, Dieppe P. Taping the patella medially: a new treatment for osteoarthritis of the knee joint? British Medical Journal 1994; 308(6931): 753–755
46. Superio-Cabuslay E, Ward MM, Lorig KR. Patient education interventions in osteoarthritis and rheumatoid arthritis: a meta-analytic comparison with nonsteroidal anti-inflammatory drug treatment. Arthritis Care and Research 1996; 9(4): 292–301
47. Felson DT, Zhang Y, Anthony JM, Naimark A, Anderson JJ. Weight loss reduces the risk for symptomatic knee osteoarthritis in women. Annals of Internal Medicine 1992; 116(7): 535–539
48. Williams RA, Foulsham BM. Weight reduction in osteoarthritis using phenteramine. Practitioner 1981; 225(1352): 231–232
49. Toda Y, Toda T, Takemura S, Wada T, Morimoto T, Ogawa R. Change in body fat, but not body weight or metabolic correlates of obesity, is related to symptomatic relief of obese patients with knee osteoarthritis after a weight control program. Journal of Rheumatology 1998; 25(11): 2181–2186
50. Bradley MH, Goulden EL. Powdered meal replacements – can they benefit overweight patients with concomitant conditions exacerbated by obesity? Current Therapeutic Research 1990; 47(3): 429–436
51. Mulrow CD, Chiquette E, Awjiel L et al. Dieting to reduce body weight for controlling hypertension in adults (Cochrane review). In: The Cochrane Library, issue 1. Oxford: Update Software, 2000
52. Creamer P. Intra-articular corticosteroid treatment in osteoarthritis. Current Opinion in Rheumatology 1999; 11(5): 417–421
53. Kirwan JR, Rankin E. Intra-articular therapy in osteoarthritis. Ballière's Clinical Rheumatology 1997; 11(4): 769–794
54. Ravaud P, Moulinier L, Giraudeau B et al. Effects of joint lavage and steroid injection in patients with osteoarthritis of the knee: results of a multicenter, randomised controlled trial. Arthritis and Rheumatism 1999; 42(3): 475–482
55. Callahan CM, Drake BG, Heck DA, Dittus RS. Patient outcomes following tri-compartmental total knee replacement: a meta-analysis. Journal of the American Medical Association 1994; 271(17): 1349–1357

56. Towheed TE, Hochberg MC. Health-related quality of life after total hip replacement. Seminars in Arthritis and Rheumatism 1996; 26(1): 483–491
57. Coventry MB, Beckenbaugh RD, Nolan DR, Ilstrup DM. 2012 total hip arthroplasties: a study of postoperative cause and early complications. Journal of Bone and Joint Surgery. American Volume 1974; 56(2): 273–284
58. White RH, McCurdy SA, Marder RA. Early morbidity after total hip replacement: rheumatoid arthritis versus osteoarthritis. Journal of General Internal Medicine 1990; 5(4): 304–309
59. Faulkner A, Kennedy LG, Baxter K, Donovan J, Wilkinson M, Bevan G. Effectiveness of hip prostheses in primary total hip replacement: a critical review of evidence and an economic model. Health Technology Assessment 1998; 2(6): 1–133
60. Young NL, Cheah D, Waddell JP, Wright JG. Patient characteristics that affect the outcome of total hip arthroplasty: a review. Canadian Journal of Surgery 1998; 41(3): 188–195

9

Acne

Sarah Purdy

Importance

Common acne (acne vulgaris) is a disease of the pilosebaceous glands and is characterised by follicular occlusion (comedones), inflammation and scars.[1] Acne occurs on the face, and also on the neck, back, chest, upper arms and buttocks. Four factors contribute to the development of acne:[2]

1. increased sebum secretion rate
2. abnormal follicular differentiation, causing obstruction of the pilosebaceous duct
3. bacteriology of the pilosebaceous duct
4. inflammation.

The anaerobic bacterium *Propionibacterium acnes* plays an important role in the pathogenesis of acne.[2] *P. acnes* releases a lipase enzyme which hydrolyses sebum triglycerides into glycerol and irritant fatty acids, which contribute to inflammation.

Acne is the most common skin disease of adolescence, affecting 80% of adolescents.[3] Androgen secretion is the major trigger for adolescent acne.[4] The number of adults over the age of 25 presenting with acne appears to be increasing; the reasons for this increase are uncertain.[5] Although acne is not associated with severe morbidity, it can have considerable psychological, social and economic consequences.[6] In severe cases, acne can lead to scarring which may exacerbate the psychosocial effects of the disease.

Review of evidence relating to indicator set

Screening

Screening patients for acne has not been recommended.

Diagnosis

Acne includes both non-inflammatory and inflammatory lesions. Non-inflammatory comedones may be open (blackhead) or closed (whitehead). Inflammatory lesions include papules, pustules, nodules or cysts. Other features are scars and hyperpigmentation. Individual patients may have one or more predominant type of lesion or a mixture of many lesions.[1,2] The following history elements have been recommended in the diagnosis of acne:[2,7]

- age at onset
- location (face, neck, chest, back, shoulders, buttocks)
- aggravating factors (e.g. seasonal, cosmetics, occupational)
- menstrual history and premenstrual worsening of acne
- family history of acne
- previous treatments, including over-the-counter therapies
- medications and drug use
- psychological and social impact.

The physical examination should include:

- location of acne
- severity and extent of disease (numbers of each types of lesion and intensity of inflammation, including hyperpigmentation and scarring).

Treatment

The main aims of treatment are to:

- reduce the number of lesions
- reduce the impact of psychological distress
- limit the duration of the disease
- prevent scarring.

The treatment chosen is dependent on an understanding of the pathology, severity, type of lesions present, patient acceptability, previous treatment and the options available.[1]

Mild acne

Mild acne consists of open and closed comedones and some papules and pustules.[1] Topical treatment is usually recommended.[1,8] The following topical treatments are available.

Benzoyl peroxide

Method of action: antibacterial and keratolytic.

Advantages:

- effective antibacterial and mild anti-inflammatory[9]
- mild anti-comedonal, especially at higher strengths[9]
- no antibiotic resistance problems
- cheap and available over the counter[8].

Disadvantages:

▶ local irritation and dermatitis (especially higher strength)[8]

▶ slow to work[1]

Topical retinoids (tretinoin, isotretinoin and adapalene)
Method of action: comedolytic.

Advantages:

▶ effective at reducing comedones[9]

▶ similar anticomedonal effect as benzoyl peroxide but less anti-inflammatory effect[8]

Disadvantages:[8,10]

▶ causes redness and peeling, usually settles with time

▶ acne may worsen for first few weeks

▶ avoid in pregnancy and breastfeeding; adequate contraception required (indicators 4 and 5)

▶ need to avoid ultra-violet light and sunlight

▶ need to allow peeling from other agents to subside before using retinoids.

Topical antibiotics
Method of action: precise mechanism unknown. Reduce numbers of *P. acnes*.[8]

Advantages:

▶ reduce inflammatory lesions

▶ less irritant than benzoyl peroxide, but no more effective.[8]

Disadvantages:

▶ antimicrobial resistance[1]

▶ tetracycline stains skin and clothing[10]

▶ contact dermatitis.[10]

Clindamycin and erythromycin have similar effectiveness.[1] Tetracycline is usually less acceptable to patients. There is evidence that combining benzoyl peroxide with topical erythromycin is more effective than topical erythromycin alone in reducing *P. acnes*. This does not appear to prevent resistance.[11]

Moderate acne
Moderate acne encompasses more frequent pustules and papules than mild acne, with mild scarring. Topical and systemic treatments are usually recommended.[1,8] The following systemic treatments are available to primary care clinicians:

Oral antibiotics
Method of action: precise mechanism unknown. Inhibit *P. acnes* and may have additional anti-inflammatory action.[2] Oral antibiotics are widely used in the management of moderate and severe acne. Drug choice depends on adverse effects, resistance, previous treatment, likely compliance and cost. Tetracyclines are considered to be the drugs of first choice.[1,2]

Tetracycline and oxytetracycline
Advantages:

▶ effective and inexpensive[2]

▶ inflammatory lesions reduced by 50% after 6 weeks.

Disadvantages:

▶ needs to be taken on an empty stomach which can affect compliance[8]

▶ gastrointestinal upsets and vaginal candidiasis are common[2]

▶ should be avoided in pregnancy, when breastfeeding and in children under the age of 12 years (indicators 1, 2 and 3)[10]

▶ can cause oral contraceptive failure during the first few weeks of treatment (indicator 3).[8]

Minocycline
A Cochrane review of the use of minocycline in acne has concluded that there is insufficient evidence to determine the comparative efficacy of minocycline relative to other acne treatments.[12] Similarly, due to inadequate research evidence, no conclusions could be drawn regarding the relative safety of minocycline.

Advantages:

▶ less likely to interact with food and milk

▶ once-daily dosage available.

Disadvantages:

▶ concerns about serious adverse effects[8,10]

▶ high cost

▶ should be avoided in pregnancy, when breastfeeding and in children under the age of 12 years[10] (indicators 1, 2 and 3)

▶ can cause oral contraceptive failure in first few weeks of treatment.[8] (indicator 3)

Doxycycline
Advantages:

▶ less likely to interact with food and milk

▶ once-daily dosage available.

Disadvantages:

▶ no benefit over tetracycline

▶ high cost

▶ should be avoided in pregnancy, when breastfeeding and in children under 12 years[10] (indicators 1, 2 and 3)

▶ can cause oral contraceptive failure during the first few weeks of treatment.[8] (indicator 3)

Erythromycin
Erythromycin has been shown to be as effective as tetracycline in the treatment of inflammatory acne. However, *P. acnes* resistance to erythromycin is common.[2]

Advantages:

▶ can be used in some patients for whom tetracyclines are not suitable.[8]

Disadvantages:

▶ antibiotic resistance

▶ gastrointestinal upset[10]

▶ can cause oral contraceptive failure during the first few weeks of treatment.

There is no evidence that combining oral antibiotics with topical benzoyl peroxide reduces bacterial resistance in *P. acnes*. Measures to minimize antibiotic resistance in acne have been suggested.[8]

Anti-androgen therapy
Method of action: reduces circulating androgens. The sebaceous gland is an androgen target organ. There is little evidence to suggest hormonal disturbance in girls with acne, but 46% of women aged 18–32 years who continue with, or develop, acne have increases in circulating testosterone.

Cyproterone acetate 2 mg and ethinyloestradiol 35 µg (Dianette) is licensed for the treatment of acne refractory to prolonged oral antibiotic therapy in female patients.

Advantages:

▶ equally effective as oral tetracycline[1]

▶ acts as contraceptive which may suit some patients.

Disadvantages:

▶ may take 3–6 months to produce beneficial effect when used alone

▶ should be withdrawn when acne is resolved – necessitating change in contraception.

A recent Cochrane review suggested that there is insufficient evidence available to determine whether spironolactone is an effective treatment for acne.[13]

It has been suggested that combined pills containing norethisterone or levonorgestrel may aggravate acne, but those with desogesterol or gestodene do not.[1] However, the latter carry an increased risk of venous thromboembolism.[10] A recent study does not support the suggestion that norethisterone or levonorgestrel may aggravate acne.[14]

Severe acne

Severe acne includes comedones, papules and pustules with scarring, plus nodular abscesses. It leads to more extensive scarring which may be keloidal in some cases. Treatment of severe acne can include the measures described for mild and moderate acne, including higher doses of tetracyclines or erythromycin.[1] However, oral retinoids are much more effective. They act by reducing sebum production. Prescription of isotretinoin requires specialist referral and monitoring of potential side-effects. Specialist referral is recommended for patients with:[3,15]

▶ severe nodular or cystic acne

▶ scarring or pigmentation

▶ poor treatment response

▶ unpleasant side-effects from current treatment

▶ severe psychological distress

▶ late-onset acne

▶ acne fulminans with systemic symptoms (requires urgent admission).

Early treatment with oral isotretinoin can reduce scarring and should be considered for the following patients:[1]

▶ severe nodular or cystic acne

▶ moderate acne resistant to conventional treatment (two courses of oral antibiotics at correct dose for correct length of time)

▶ acne of late onset in mid-20s or 30s (often less responsive to oral antibiotics).

Adverse reactions to oral isotretinoin are common. Management should include the following:[10]

▶ exclude pregnancy prior to starting treatment

▶ adequate contraception including 1 month before and after treatment

▶ check plasma lipids and liver function tests before treatment, 1 month after treatment commences, then 3-monthly

▶ counsel the patient regarding side-effects and the need to avoid blood donation and wax epilation.

Other techniques for treating severe acne, such as local steroid injection, are used by dermatologists.[2] There is currently insufficient evidence about the effectiveness of laser treatment for acne scarring.[16,17]

Advice and counselling

Diet and poor skin cleansing do not worsen acne.[18] Indeed, abrasive cleansers and vigorous cleaning may worsen acne by increasing inflammation. Patients should be involved in the choice of treatment and therapies should be acceptable to patients. Topical treatments must be cosmetically acceptable. Gels and solutions are generally more suitable for oily skin, but may sting. Creams are more suitable for dry or sensitive skin. Lotions are suitable for large or hairy areas.[8,10] It is important that patients understand how to use their treatment and are aware of common side-effects. The likely time scale for improvement and duration of treatment should be explained. Primary care clinicians have a large part to play in counselling and supporting patients with acne. Psychological stress is common and acne can affect patients' employment prospects and social life, with consequent psychological effects.[1,6]

Follow-up

Topical agents generally require at least 2 months of treatment before improvement occurs. Treatment should be reassessed every 2–3 months and continued until improvement occurs. The definition of successful treatment should take into account the patient's expectations. Improvement has been defined as a situation where no further lesions are developing.[18]

Recommended quality indicators for acne

Treatment
1 Oral tetracycline should not be prescribed for children under 12 years of age
2 If oral tetracycline is prescribed for a female of childbearing age (16–45 years), enquiry should be made about the date of last menstrual period or a negative pregnancy test
3 If oral tetracycline is prescribed for a female of childbearing age (16–45 years), advice should be given regarding effective means of contraception (including abstinence)
4 If topical retinoids are prescribed to females of childbearing age (16–45 years), enquiry should be made about the date of last menstrual period or a negative pregnancy test
5 If topical retinoids are prescribed to females of childbearing age (16–45 years), advice should be given regarding effective means of contraception (including abstinence)

A response to oral antibiotics is usually seen after 3 months, although it may take 6 months for maximum response. Some patients may need to take them for 2 years or more. An adequate dose of oral antibiotic should be given for at least 3 months before deciding that a patient has failed to respond.[2]

Overview of data sources used in this review

A literature search was conducted using the Medline, Cochrane Library and NHS Centre for Reviews and Dissemination databases. Search parameters on Medline were acne vulgaris, 1990 to August 2000, limited to English language. Searches for reviews of acne treatment were conducted on the other databases. Searches were scanned for relevant systematic reviews and randomised controlled trials. Relevant papers were obtained and reviewed. The reference lists of papers were searched for other key references. One leading UK expert in the field of acne was consulted regarding the review and the authors of the registered Cochrane and HTA protocols were contacted regarding their work.

Good-quality data from randomised controlled trials with objective outcome measures are lacking for many treatments used in acne. Two Cochrane reviews were identified: one covered a specialist therapeutic area (spironolactone plus or minus steroids in the treatment of hirsutism and acne); the other is included in this discussion.[12,13] No other existing reviews that follow a rigorous systematic methodology were identified. There is a protocol registered for one other relevant Cochrane review and the British Association of Dermatology is aiming to produce evidence-based guidelines for the treatment of acne later in 2000 (W.J. Cunliffe, personal communication).[19] One large randomised parallel group trial of antibiotics for acne is in progress.[20] One review of the broad issues in acne management was available.[8] This was systematic in nature but would not meet criteria for a full systematic review.

Acknowledgements

I would like to thank Professor W.J. Cunliffe, Samantha Lane of the National Prescribing Centre and Julie Glanville of the NHS Centre for Reviews and Dissemination.

Further reading

Brown SK, Shalita AR. Acne vulgaris. Lancet 1998; 351: 1871–1876

Cunliffe WJ. Management of adult acne and acne variants. Journal of Cutaneous Medicine and Surgery 1998; 2(s3): 7–13

Darvay A, Chu A. Pocket guide to acne. Oxford: Blackwell, 2000

References

1. Healy E, Simpson N. Acne vulgaris. British Medical Journal 1994; 308: 831–833
2. Brown SK, Shalita AR. Acne vulgaris. Lancet 1998; 351: 1871–1876
3. Chu TC. Acne and other facial eruptions. Medicine 1997; 25: 30–33
4. Webster GF. Acne vulgaris: state of the science. Archives of Dermatology 1999; 135(9): 1101–1102
5. Cunliffe WJ. Management of adult acne and acne variants. Journal of Cutaneous Medicine and Surgery 1998; 2(s3): 7–13
6. Mallon E, Newton JN, Klassen A et al. The quality of life in acne: a comparison with general medical conditions using generic questionnaires. British Journal of Dermatology 1999; 140(4): 672–676
7. Darvay A, Chu A. Pocket guide to acne. Oxford: Blackwell, 2000
8. National Prescribing Centre. The treatment of acne vulgaris: an update. MeReC Bulletin 1999; 10 (8): 29–32
9. Gollnick H, Schramm M. Topical drug treatment in acne. Dermatology 1998; 196: 119–125
10. British National Formulary. March 2000. London: BMJ
11. Eady EA, Bojar RA, Jones CE et al. The effects of acne treatment with a combination of benzoyl peroxide and erythromycin on skin carriage of erythromycin-resistant bacteria. British Journal of Dermatology 1996; 134: 107–113
12. Garner SE, Eady EA, Li Wan Po A, Newton J, Popescu C. Minocycline for acne vulgaris: efficacy and safety. The Cochrane Library, Issue 1. Oxford: Update Software, 2000

13. Lee O, Farquhar C, Toomath R, Jepson R. Spironolactone versus placebo or in combination with steroids for hirsutism and/or acne. The Cochrane Library, issue 4. Oxford: Update Software, 1999

14. Thorneycroft IH, Stanczyk FZ, Bradshaw KD et al. Effect of low dose oral contraceptives on androgenic markers and acne. Contraception 1999; 60(5): 255–262

15. Russell-Jones R. Guidelines for GP referrals in dermatology. Beckenham: Publishing Initiatives, 1996

16. Jordan R, Cummins C, Burls A. Laser resurfacing of the skin for the improvement of facial acne scarring. The Cochrane Library, issue 1. Oxford: Update Software, 2000

17. Jordan R, Cummins C, Burls A. Laser resurfacing of the skin for the improvement of facial acne scarring: a systematic review of the evidence. British Journal of Dermatology 2000; 142(3): 413–423

18. Leyden JJ. Therapy for acne vulgaris. New England Journal of Medicine 1997; 336: 1157–1162

19. Coates P, Eady AE, Cove JH. Complementary therapies for acne (protocol for a Cochrane Review). The Cochrane Library, Issue 1. Oxford: Update Software, 2000

20. UK NHS National Coordinating Centre for Technology Assessment. Identification of the most cost effective, microbiologically safe antimicrobial treatments for acne. NCCHTA (expected date of publication mid-2002).

▶10

Acute low back pain

Martin Underwood

Importance

Low back pain has a large health and social impact. Invalidity Benefit paid for chronic spinal disorders increased by 226% in the UK in the 10 years to 1994. There has since been a modest fall, coincident with benefit regulation changes.[1] The prevalence of back pain appears unchanged,[2] suggesting that there is an epidemic of back pain disability rather than an epidemic of back pain. A reported increase in prevalence is thought to result from changed awareness of symptoms and willingness to report symptoms rather than an actual increase.[3]

One in 6 people report having back pain on any day, 1 in 3 in the last month and 6% long-standing or serious disabling low back pain in the previous year.[4] Around 60–80% of the population report previous back pain.[5] The true incidence may be even higher because of recall bias. Around 5–10% of those presenting with new episodes of back pain develop chronic problems. These individuals account for the majority of the costs of back pain.[2] Back pain was estimated to cost the UK £5000 million in 1998:[6] £1067 million in NHS costs; £565 million in other health care costs and £3440 million in indirect costs such as lost production.

Building on a Clinical Standards Advisory Group report,[2] the Royal College of General Practitioners produced acute back pain guidelines in 1997, which were revised in 1999.[7] Back pain patients who do not have nerve root compression or reasons to suspect a serious underlying condition should be classified as having 'simple back pain' and be encouraged to resume normal activity as soon as possible.

Review of evidence relating to indicator set

Screening and primary prevention

Seven of 11 epidemiological studies reviewed by Lahad[8] found that fitness or flexibility was associated with reduced low back pain. Two further studies also suggest that physical activity protects against the development of back pain[9,10] and one[11] that physical activity outside work did not increase risk of back pain. A systematic review of intervention studies found some evidence that exercise may prevent back pain in occupational settings.[12] One of 5 of occupational studies of education found a reduction in back pain. Three of the remaining studies had medium-term positive outcomes and all 4 had long-term negative outcomes.[8] A systematic review found moderate evidence that lumbar supports are ineffective in preventing back pain.[13]

Smoking, obesity and psychological factors are associated with back pain. There are other reasons for modifying these factors but no evidence to support their use for preventing back pain.[8,14,15] No specific evidence-based recommendations were agreed on the prevention of acute back pain.

Diagnosis

The national acute low back pain guidelines[7] recommend diagnostic triage of patients with acute back pain into four groups:

1. *Simple backache*

   ▶ presenting age 29–55 years

   ▶ lumbosacral, buttocks and thighs

   ▶ 'mechanical' pain

   ▶ patient well

2. *Nerve root pain*

   ▶ unilateral leg pain worse than low back pain

   ▶ radiates to foot or toes

   ▶ numbness and paraesthesia in same distribution

   ▶ straight leg raise (SLR) reproduces leg pain

   ▶ localised neurological signs

3. *Red flags for* possible *serious spinal pathology* (indicator 1)

   ▶ presentation under the age of 20 or onset over 55 years

   ▶ non-mechanical pain

   ▶ thoracic pain

   ▶ past history: carcinoma, steroids, HIV

   ▶ unwell, weight loss

   ▶ Widespread neurological symptoms or signs

   ▶ structural deformity

4. *Cauda equina syndrome* (indicator 2)

   ▶ sphincter disturbance (bladder or bowels)

   ▶ gait disturbance

   ▶ saddle anaesthesia.

A review of the accuracy of history, physical examination and erythrocyte sedimentation rate (ESR) in the diagnosis of back pain in general practice[16] found that the specificity and sensitivity of symptoms and signs was not great in the diagnosis of nerve root compression or vertebral cancer. The combination of a suggestive clinical history (age >50, unexplained weight loss, previous history of cancer, failure of medical treatment) and a raised ESR was valuable in the diagnosis of malignancy.

The 'red flags' are therefore indications for considering further investigation. They do not mean that any individual who has one or more of these must have additional investigation[1] (indicator 1).

Bigos et al.[17] considered the use of x-rays in the diagnosis of back pain. They found moderate research evidence that plain x-rays are not recommended for the routine evaluation of patients with acute low back problems within the first month unless a red flag is present. Arranging x-rays of the lumbar spine may adversely affect patient outcome and increase general practitioner workload[18] (indicator 3). National guidelines recommend that initial assessment should include:

▶ The patient's age, the duration and description of symptoms, the impact of symptoms on activity and work, and the response to previous therapy.

▶ Psychological or socioeconomic problems in the individual's life since such factors can complicate both assessment and treatment.

▶ SLR should be assessed and recorded in young adults with sciatica. In older patients with spinal stenosis, SLR may be normal.

▶ Examination for neurological abnormalities should emphasise ankle and knee reflexes, ankle and great toe dorsiflexion strength, and distribution of sensory complaints.

▶ The initial clinical history should identify 'red flags' of possible serious spinal pathology. Such inquiries are especially important in patients over the age of 50 (indicator 1).

▶ Symptoms and signs of cauda equina syndrome, widespread neurological involvement, and severe or progressive weakness are 'red flags' for severe neurological risk (indicator 2).

▶ A history of significant trauma relative to age (e.g. a fall from a height or motor vehicle accident in a young adult or a minor fall or heavy lift in a potentially osteoporotic or older person) raises the question of possible fracture (indicator 1).

The National Institute for Clinical Excellence's[19] draft guide for referral from general to specialist services suggests that patients:

▶ with features of cauda equina syndrome or if serious spinal pathology is suspected, be referred and seen immediately (indicator 1)

▶ who develop progressive neurological deficit or have nerve root pain that is not resolving after 6 weeks be referred and seen urgently, probably within 2 weeks

▶ who have simple back pain and have not resumed their normal activities in 3 months or in whom ankylosing spondylitis is suspected, be referred and seen soon.

Ankylosing spondylitis is a cause of chronic, not acute, back pain. New cases are uncommon in primary care.[20]

Psychosocial factors in developing chronic back pain

One of the goals in treating acute back pain is prevention of chronic disability.[2] Psychosocial and economic factors play an important role in chronic back pain and influence the patient's response to treatment. No randomised controlled trial data exist to demonstrate if psychosocial assessment or interventions affect the outcome of acute back pain.[7]

Treatment

Symptom education

There is evidence to suggest that appropriate information and advice can reduce anxiety and improve satisfaction with care. Appropriate advice includes:

▶ Most severe back pain/disability improves considerably in a few days or weeks. Milder symptoms frequently persist for several months.

▶ Most patients will have recurrences at some time.

▶ The longer someone is off work the lower their chance of returning to work.

▶ Back pain becomes slightly less common after the age of 50 60 years. However, older patients with back pain may have more persistent symptoms.

▶ About 10% of patients will have pain after 1 year. Patients who continue normal activities feel healthier, use fewer analgesics and are less distressed than those who limit their activities.

This advice is based on observational data. It does not show that giving any or all of this advice to patients improves outcome.

Medication

Regular paracetamol, paracetamol-weak opioid compounds, non-steroidal anti-inflammatory drugs (NSAIDs) or muscle relaxants (diazepam, baclofen, dantrolene) are all effective in reducing acute back pain.[7] Strong opioids appear to be no more effective than paracetamol, paracetamol-weak opioid compounds or NSAIDs and may have significant adverse effects including drowsiness and physical dependence.[17]

▶ NSAIDs prescribed at regular intervals effectively reduce simple backache (it is unclear whether they are more effective than simple analgesics or other drugs.[13]

▶ There is no evidence to suggest that some NSAIDs are more effective than others. They may have serious side-effects. Ibuprofen and diclofenac appear to have the lowest risk of gastrointestinal complications (there are at present insufficient data to comment on safety and efficacy of selective Cox-2 inhibitors).

▶ Muscle relaxants effectively reduce acute back pain. They may have significant side-effects, including drowsiness. There is potential for physical dependence after relatively short courses.

▶ Paracetamol or paracetamol-weak opioid compounds prescribed at regular intervals effectively reduce simple backache. Paracetamol-weak opioid compounds may be effective when NSAIDs or paracetamol alone do not provide sufficient pain control.

▶ There are no studies of the use of antidepressants for acute back pain.

Physical treatments

Manipulation
There are many controlled trials of manipulation. Systematic reviews of these have reached different conclusions.[7] Of 12 randomised controlled trials identified that included only patients with acute back pain, 5 reported positive results, 4 negative results and 3 positive results in a subgroup of the population.[21] A further trial of osteopathy was inconclusive.[22]

There is little evidence on the use of manipulation for those who have nerve root pain. However, for back pain with no nerve root symptoms the risks of manipulation are low, provided that patients are selected and assessed properly and the manipulation is carried out by a trained therapist or practitioner. In such cases manipulation provides better short-term improvement in pain, activity levels and patient satisfaction than the treatments to which it has been compared.

Other physical treatments
There is little evidence to support the use of:

▶ physical agents (ice, heat, shortwave diathermy, massage, ultrasound)

▶ traction

▶ transcutaneous electrical nerve stimulation (TENS)

▶ shoe insoles and shoe lifts

▶ lumbar corsets and supports

▶ trigger point and ligamentous injections

▶ acupuncture

▶ epidural steroid injections (for patients who also have nerve root pain they do appear to produce better short-term results than the treatments to which they have been compared)

▶ facet joint injections

▶ biofeedback

▶ massage (one paper does suggest some benefit from massage for subacute back pain[23]).

Bedrest or staying active

A number of controlled trials have considered the use of bedrest and advice to stay active for acute low back pain with or without leg pain. There is little evidence on the efficacy of bedrest for patients with nerve root pain or disc prolapse. The trials of advice regarding bedrest and activity appear to have consistent results.[7] It is therefore suggested that:

► Advice to continue ordinary activity can give equivalent or faster symptomatic recovery from an acute attack and lead to less chronic disability and less time off work than 'traditional' treatment with analgesics as required, advice to rest, allowing level to guide returning to normal activity.

► Bedrest for 2–7 days for patients with acute or recurrent low back pain is worse than placebo or ordinary activity. It is not as effective as the treatments to which it has been compared.

► Graded reactivation over a short period of days or weeks, combined with behavioural management of pain, makes little difference to the rate of initial recovery but leads to less chronic disability and work loss.

► Prolonged bedrest may lead to debilitation, chronic disability and difficulty in rehabilitation.

► Advice to return to normal work within a planned short term may lead to shorter periods of work loss and less time off work.

Exercise therapy

There are over 39 randomised controlled trials of exercise therapy for low back pain. Twelve of these with over 2000 randomised participants compared exercise therapy with either another active treatment (8) or an inactive or 'placebo' treatment (4) for patients with acute low back pain. Only one reported better outcomes in the intervention group.[13] It is therefore doubtful that specific back exercises produce clinically significant improvement in acute low back pain, or that it is possible to select which patients will respond to exercises. One study that recruited patients with back pain of 4 weeks to 6 months duration from primary care found a small but statistically significant benefit from exercise classes.[24] There is therefore some evidence that exercise programmes and physical reconditioning can improve pain and functional levels in patients with chronic low back pain in a primary care setting and there are theoretical arguments for commencing exercise programmes and physical reconditioning at around 6 weeks.

Surgery

The primary rationale for surgery for disc prolapse is to relieve nerve root irritation or compression due to herniated disc material. Chemonucleolysis with chymopapain has been compared to placebo and surgical treatment. It produced better results than placebo and worse than surgical discectomy.[25] The reviewers concluded that discectomy is more effective for carefully selected patients with sciatica due to lumbar disc prolapse than conservative treatment. In particular it provides faster relief from an acute attack, although effects on lifetime natural history of the condition are still unclear.

Treatments not recommended

The national guidelines found no evidence of benefit, or unacceptable risk:benefit ratios for the following treatments:

- narcotics for more than 2 weeks

- benzodiazepines for more than 2 weeks

- colchicine

- systemic steroids

- bedrest with traction

- manipulation under general anaesthesia

- plaster jacket.

Special diagnostic tests

In the presence of 'red flags', especially for tumour or infection, the use of bone scan, CT or MRI may be indicated even if plain x-rays are normal. A bone scan is recommended when spinal tumour, infection or occult fracture is suspected from 'red flags' on medical history, physical examination, corroborative lab. test or plain x-ray findings.

Follow-up

There are no clear indications for routine follow-up of acute low back pain.

Recommended quality indicators for acute back pain

Diagnosis
1 Patients aged 50+ presenting with sudden-onset low back pain (onset <24 hours) should be asked about a history suggestive of spinal fracture (past history of trauma, prolonged steroids, cancer, risk factors of osteoporosis)
2 Patients with referred leg pain (not buttock) should be asked about urinary disturbance

Treatment
3 X-rays should not be performed in acute lower back pain of less than 6 weeks duration unless 'red flag' signs/symptoms exist

---

Overview of data sources used in this review

A number of reviews informed this chapter.[2,7,13,17] Where there is disagreement between experts, the UK national guidelines[7] are taken as the definitive interpretation of the evidence. To ensure consistency, many of the evidence statements are the same as, or similar to, UK guidelines.

Further reading

Waddell G, Feder G, McIntosh A, Lewis M, Hutchinson A. Low back pain evidence review. London: Royal College of General Practitioners, 1999. Also available at http://www.rcgp.org.uk/college/activity/qualclin/guides/backpain/index.htm

Waddell G. The back pain revolution. London: Churchill Livingstone, 1998

References

1. DSS Figures
2. Clinical Standards Advisory Group. Epidemiological review: the epidemiology and cost of back pain. In: The annex to the CSAG report on back pain. London: HMSO, 1994
3. Palmer KT, Walsh K, Bendall H, Cooper C, Coggon D. Back pain in Britain: comparison of two prevalence surveys at an interval of 10 years. British Medical Journal 2000; 320(7249): 1577–1578
4. Croft P, Papageorgiou A, McNally R. Low back pain. In: Stevens A & Raftery J, eds. Low back pain in health care needs assessment: the epidemiologically based needs assessment reviews. Oxford: Radcliffe, 1997
5. Andersson GBJ. The epidemiology of spinal disorders. In: Frymoyer JW, ed. The adult spine: principles and practice. New York: Raven Press, 1991
6. Maniadakis N, Gray A. The economic burden of back pain in the UK. Pain 2000; 84(1): 95–103
7. Waddell G, Feder G, McIntosh A, Lewis M, Hutchinson A. Low back pain evidence review. London: Royal College of General Practitioners, 1999. Also available at http://www.rcgp.org.uk/college/activity/qualclin/guides/backpain/index.htm
8. Lahad A, Malter AD, Berg AO, Deyo RA. The effectiveness of four interventions for the prevention of low back pain. Journal of the American Medical Association 1994; 272(16): 1286–1291
9. Leino PI. Does leisure time physical activity prevent low back disorders? Spine 1993; 18(7): 863–871
10. Harreby M, Hesseøe G, Kjer J, Neergaard K. Low back pain and physical exercise in leisure time in 38-year-old women: a 25-year cohort study. European Spine Journal 1997; 6(3): 181–186
11. Croft PR, Papageorgiou AC, Thomas E, Macfarlane GJ, Silman AJ. Short-term physical risk factors for new episodes of low back pain. Spine 1999; 24(15): 1556–1561
12. van Poppell MNM, Koes BW, Smid T, Bouter LM. A systematic review of controlled clinical trials on the prevention of back pain in industry. Occupational and Environmental Medicine 1997; 54(12): 841–847
13. van Tulder MW, Koes BW, Assendelft WJJ, Bouter LM. The effectiveness of conservative treatment of acute and chronic low back pain. Amsterdam: EMGO-Instituut, 1999
14. Deyo RA, Bass JE. Lifestyle and low-back pain: the influence of smoking and obesity. Spine 1989, 14(5), 501–506
15. Leboeuf-Yde C. Smoking and low back pain. A systematic literature review of 41 journal articles reporting 47 epidemiologic studies. Spine 1999; 24(14), 1463–1470
16. van den Hoogen HMM, Koes BW, van Eijk JTM, Bouter I. On the accuracy of history, physical examination, and erythrocyte sedimentation rate in diagnosing low back pain in general practice. A criteria based literature review. Spine 1995; 20(3): 318–327
17. Bigos S, Bowyer O, Braen G et al. Acute low back problems in adults: clinical practice: guideline no. 14. Rockville, MD: Agency for Health Care Policy and Research, Public Health Service, US Department of Health and Human Services, 1994
18. Kendrick D, Fielding K, Bentley E, Kerslake R, Miller P, Pringle M. Radiography of the lumbar spine in primary care patients with low back pain: randomised controlled trial. BMJ 2001; 322(7283): 400–405
19. National Institute for Clinical Excellence. Referral practice, a guide to appropriate referral from general to specialist services. Version under pilot. London: NICE, 2000. Also available at http://www.nice.org.uk/nice-web/pdf/NICEGPReferralcues4.pdf
20. Underwood MR, Dawes P. Inflammatory back pain in primary care. British Journal of Rheumatology 1995; 34(11): 1074–1077
21. Koes BW, Assendelft WJJ, van der Heijden G, Bouter LM. Spinal manipulation for low back pain. An updated systematic review of randomised controlled trials. Spine 1996; 21(24): 2860–2871
22. Andersson GBJ, Lucente T, Davis AM, Kappler RE, Lipton JA, Leurgans S. A comparison of osteopathic manipulation with standard care for patients with low back pain. New England Journal of Medicine 1999; 341(19): 1426–1431

23.   Preyde M. Effectiveness of massage therapy for subacute low-back pain: a randomized controlled trial. Canadian Medical Association Journal 2000; 162(13): 1815–1820

24.   Moffett JK, Torgerson D, Bell-Syer S et al. Randomised controlled trial of exercise for low back pain: clinical outcomes, costs and preferences. British Medical Journal 1999; 319(7205): 279–283

25.   Gibson JNA, Grant IC, Waddell G. Surgery for lumbar disc prolapse (Cochrane review) The Cochrane Library, issue 3, Oxford: Update Software, 2000

▶11

Acute diarrhoea in children

Pali Hungin

Importance

Acute diarrhoeal disease is one of the most common presenting conditions in children. The RCGP Morbidity Statistics from General Practice (1991–2)[1] indicate the following disease and consultation rates for intestinal infections in the 0–4 and 5–15 age groups (Tables 11.1 and 11.2).

The immediate potential problem associated with acute gastroenteritis is dehydration. The basic remit of the GP is to assess the child presenting with acute diarrhoea with regard to hydration status (indicators 3, 4 and 5), fluid intake and the risk of generalised infection, to institute home management where appropriate, and to determine whether hospital treatment should be considered.[2-4]

Less than 50% of those with acute diarrhoea are estimated as presenting to the GP and less than 5% of these are admitted to hospital. The aetiology of acute diarrhoea is formally established in a very small proportion and laboratory data on pathogens are based on the estimated <1% in which investigations are done. The reported aetiology is therefore likely to be biased. The commonest cause of acute diarrhoea is viral and it is generally self-limiting, without complications.

Table 11.1 Specific pathogens

	0–4 years	5–15 years
Salmonella	12	2
Shigellosis	8	6
Other bacterial food poisoning	1	1
Protozoal disease	5	2
Other organisms	26	7

Table 11.2 Ill-defined infections

	0–4 years	5–15 years
Incidence	2011	387
Prevalence	1827	379
Consultation	2541	428

All expressed as rates per 10 000 person years at risk

The incidence is highest among children aged 1–3 years[5] and among those attending care facilities. By extrapolation of RCGP data and laboratory reports the PHLS Communicable Disease Centre[6] estimated that rotavirus alone accounted for 762 000 new episodes of infectious intestinal disease in children under the age of 5 years, between 1992 and 1996[7] in England and Wales. Despite the relatively high prevalence of acute diarrhoea in children the death rate in the UK is low, though there are no specific current data available. Death is usually related to complications such as dehydration, electrolyte abnormalities and shock, and occurs mostly in infants under 1 year old.[5] Particular care is required when managing children under the age of 3 years.

Review of evidence relating to indicator set

Screening and prevention

Screening is not appropriate but clinicians should be aware of the higher risk of infection in those attending childcare facilities and in those who are immunocompromised. Breastfeeding offers some protection but prevention through immunisation is unlikely to be in clinical use in Europe in the immediate future.[8]

Diagnosis

The severity of illness of those presenting with a history of diarrhoea, defined by DeWitt[9] as stools abnormally frequent or liquid, should be determined (indicator 1). This includes the duration, the consistency and character and the frequency of stools. Assessment should include the intake of fluids and urinary output[9,10] and the possibility of fever, abdominal pain, tenesmus, vomiting,[9,11] antibiotic use and contact with persons with similar symptoms. If available, the stool should be examined, especially for presence of gross blood.[11]

An assessment of the child's hydration status is paramount.[12] This is because the electrolyte and hydration imbalances occurring in acute diarrhoea, together with systemic infection, are responsible for much of the associated morbidity and mortality, especially in those under the age of 3 years (indicators 1, 2 and 5).

The clinical signs of dehydration are usually absent in children with less than 5% dehydration and thirst and decreased urine output may be the only pointers[2] (indicators 3 and 4). The possibility of septicaemia must also be considered, particularly in infants and in the presence of fever and blood in the stool.[13,14]

Causative agents

The commonest cause of acute diarrhoea in children is viral infection (80%), followed by bacterial and protozoal infections. The commonest virus is the rotavirus. It is thought to spread by the fecal-oral and respiratory routes.[11,13,15] Of 160 000 reports of fecal pathogen identifications from children under the age of 5 years in England and Wales between 1992 and 1996 the Public Health Laboratory Service reported that 43% were due to rotavirus. In two-thirds of children the diarrhoea is preceded by a respiratory illness. Rotavirus is rarely detected in children over the age of 6 years, by which age most have developed antibodies. Those aged 6–18 months are the most susceptible and rotavirus infection is commonest during the winter, when it is the main cause of acute diarrhoea in children. The incubation period is 1–3 days with viral excretion at its highest during the third and fourth days and virtually complete viral clearance by the eighth day. An attack of rotavirus infection appears to confer immunity against further episodes.

Norwalk viruses, resembling rotaviruses, are less common but also occur in the winter. Infection is usually from a common source and is characterised by family or community outbreaks.[16] In contrast to rotavirus, Norwalk infections are commoner in those over the age of 6 years. The incubation period is 1–2 days with symptoms persisting for 3 days or so. Immunity develops only slowly and adults may also be affected.

Enteric adenoviruses can also cause acute diarrhoea, especially in children aged 2 years and under.[13] The incubation period is 10 days with an illness lasting for 5–12 days.[11,13] Infection is usually by the fecal-oral[16] or person-to-person route. Other less common viruses include pestivirus, astrovirus, calicivirus, parvovirus and non-group A rotavirus.[17]

Bacterial causes of acute diarrhoea are less common. The incidence of 'dysentery' as listed by the Public Health Laboratory Service is declining in the UK with notifications having dropped from 9935 in 1991 to 1813 in 1998.[6] Salmonella is the commonest bacterial cause of diarrhoea and infants younger than 6 months are especially susceptible. It is acquired through contaminated foods, particularly meat, dairy and poultry products.[11] The incubation period is 2–3 days and the duration of illness 2–3 days. Shigella, transmitted from person to person, is the second most common bacterial cause of acute diarrhoea among children aged 6 months to 10 years but is uncommon in infants under 6 months of age.[17]

Table 11.3 World Health Organization factors for assessing hydration status

	Degree of hydration		
Factors	Minimal	Mild to moderate	Severe
General condition	Well, alert	*Restless, irritable	*Lethargic or unconscious, floppy
Eyes	Normal	Sunken	Very sunken and dry
Tears	Present	Absent	Absent
Mouth and tongue	Moist	Dry	Very dry
Thirst	Drinks normally, not thirsty	*Thirsty, drinks eagerly	* Drinks poorly or not able to drink
Skin pinch	Skin goes back quickly	*Skin goes back slowly	*Skin goes back very slowly
Decision	No signs of dehydration	*2 or more of the above signs including at least one 'key' sign	*2 or more of the above signs, including at least one 'key' sign

* key sign of dehydration
Mild dehydration: 50–100 ml/kg estimated fluid deficit
Severe dehydration: >100 ml/kg fluid deficit[12]

Campylobacter is most frequent among children and young adults.[16] Public Health Laboratory Service data for 1998 for the UK indicate 6157 positive laboratory reports for the 0–4 age group and 3816 for the 5–14 age group. Incubation is 1–7 days and transmission is commonly by the fecal-oral route.[16]

Bacteria can cause enterotoxigenic diarrhoea. Some toxins are ingested while others are produced in the intestine. Ingestion of toxin in cases of *S. aureus* or *B. cereus* lead to a brief duration of diarrhoea after an incubation period of 1–6 hours.[11] *C. perfringens*, found in contaminated foods, causes a 3-day bout of severe diarrhoea following an 8- to 12-hour incubation period.[11] *C. difficile* is associated with antibiotic use and can cause pseudomembranous colitis and may spread from patient to patient.[11] There has been a steady increase in cholera notifications in the UK, from 22 to 48 between 1991 and 1998.[6] *Giardia*, the commonest parasitic cause, is also detected occasionally.[17]

Conditions that may masquerade as acute gastroenteritis[2]

Surgical:

▶ pyloric stenosis

▶ intususseception

▶ acute appendicitis

Medical:

▶ systemic infections

▶ otitis media

▶ coeliac disease

▶ cow's milk protein intolerance

▶ adrenal insufficiency

▶ Reye's syndrome.

Clinical pattern

Distinguishing between viral and bacterial infection on clinical grounds is not reliable. Blood or mucus in the stool suggests an enteroinvasive pathogen, while vomiting preceded by prodromal upper respiratory tract symptoms and followed by watery diarrhoea suggests rotavirus.[2]

Laboratory diagnosis

Microscopic examination of stool and cultures may be warranted where public health intervention is required.[18] It may also be helpful for children who have an inflammatory clinical pattern of acute diarrhoea with bloody stools and fever,[9,13,18] especially when diarrhoea persists for more than 3 days.[11] Those with symptoms lasting longer than 10–14 days may warrant stool examination for ova and para-sites,[9,11] *Giardia* may be diagnosed by direct microscopic examination of stool specimens.

Treatment

Fluid and electrolyte correction

Most episodes of acute diarrhoea require only fluid and electrolyte stabilisation and feeding therapy without other intervention.[9,11,19,20]

Oral rehydration therapy in children with mild-to-moderate dehydration consists of replacement of the fluid deficit and ongoing losses and the provision of mainte-nance fluid, electrolyte and nutritional needs. If the child is not yet dehydrated, maintenance of the regular diet and the early initiation of oral hydration therapy at home with a carbohydrate-electrolyte solution (20–50 mcq/L of sodium per litre) is recommended.[10,11,21] If electrolyte solutions are not available then soups, unsweet-ened fruit juices, yoghurt-based drinks and plain water with starchy foods contain-ing some salt may be used. Those unable to tolerate fluids should be admitted to hospital.

In mild-to-moderate dehydration, oral fluid deficit replacement should occur over the initial 4–5 hours in a supervised setting, usually in hospital.[10–12,16,21] Vomiting is not an absolute contraindication to oral rehydration with the volume increased as tolerated.[10,16,18,21] Non-breast fed infants under 6 months of age should be given 100–200 ml of additional water during the rehydration phase, while breast-fed infants should continue breast feeding.[18]

Sihal & Booth[2] suggest the following indicators suggesting consideration of hospital admission:

▶ age less than 6 months

▶ profuse vomiting or diarrhoea

▶ clinically detectable dehydration

▶ severe systemic symptoms

▶ pre-existing medical illness predisposing to dehydration (e.g. diabetes, ileostomy)

▶ diagnostic uncertainty

▶ unfavourable home circumstances.

Feeding during the illness (refeeding)

The issue of refeeding, particularly in infants, has been controversial[22] and current guidelines are only patchily applied.[23] In the UK it has sometimes been the practice to cease breast milk, formula or milk and solids until after the initial 24 hours of glucose-electrolyte solution therapy. The ESPGAN Working Group[19] on acute diarrhoea reiterated that successful management of gastroenteritis relies chiefly on the maintenance or restoration of adequate rehydration and electrolyte balance together with maintenance of adequate nutritional intake. They support refeeding during oral rehydration on the basis that early feeding may decrease intestinal permeability induced by infection and may lead to better gut healing and maintenance of disaccharidase activity. An ESPGAN multicentre trial[3] and UK-based work[24] showed that early feeding resulted in significant weight gain compared with late feeding and did not result in worsening or prolongation of diarrhoea, vomiting or lactose intolerance. The continuation of breast feeding is also endorsed by the ESPGAN guidelines.[19]

The use of formula milk

Children on milk-based formulas may continue with smaller, more frequent feeds or diluted cereals and other foods. The ESPGAN guidelines[19] endorse this, pointing out that adverse outcomes are more likely when patients have had severe dehydration or previous therapy failures. A normal lactose-containing diet is recommended in most cases. However, if the diarrhoea worsens on the reintroduction of milk, stool pH and/or reducing substances should be checked and lactose content reduced if intolerance is suggested.

Some clinicians advocate lactose-free formulas for children with acute diarrhoea.[25] It was concluded from a meta-analysis of trials[25] that the routine use of lactose-free milk formula was not warranted since the increased duration of diarrhoea with lactose-containing formula was not clinically significant. The ESPGAN advice echoes this. The routine dilution of formula is not necessary.

Solids and semi-solids during the illness

These should be continued during the diarrhoeal episode, particularly easily digestible, high-calorie items which can include eggs and dairy products, mashed cooked vegetables and bananas and starches. Studies have shown that the duration of diarrhoea is markedly reduced in those receiving staple foods.[18,22]

Drug therapy

In viral diarrhoea, hydration is the mainstay of treatment whether it is oral or parenteral, and specific drugs are not available.

Few of those with bacterial diarrhoea are likely to benefit from antibiotics. Empirical antibiotic treatment is not indicated in non-toxic infants with acute diarrhoea (indicator 6). Antibiotics should not be used unless there is a positive diagnosis and the child is not improving. The BNF[26] recommendations for antibiotics, when required, are trimethoprim or ciproflaxin for Salmonella, although this may prolong the period of fecal shedding of the organism[18] and increase the risk of the asymptomatic carrier state;[16] trimethoprim or ciproflaxin for shigellosis. For Campylobacter, antibiotic therapy (erythromycin or ciproflaxin[26]) may only be effective early in the illness[18] and is used in epidemic situations or if severe fever or bloody diarrhoea is present.[11]

Confirmed Giardia, in the presence of symptoms over 2 weeks, responds to metronidazole, tinidazole or mepacrine[26] and amoebiasis to metronidazole or tinidazole.[26]

Antidiarrhoeals and antimotility drugs

Antimotility agents or adsorbents should not be used for the treatment of acute diarrhoea in children.[9–11,18,27–30] Most are not approved for children and have been shown to be ineffective in trials.[18] Antimotility medications can worsen the clinical course in shigellosis and in antibiotic-associated colitis.[31]

Follow-up

Young infants and those with severe diarrhoea are more likely to fail to respond to treatment.[22] Those with diarrhoea for longer than 14 days should be investigated for causes of persistent or chronic diarrhoea.[11,19]

Recommended quality indicators for acute diarrhoea in children

Diagnosis

1 Children under 16 years presenting with acute diarrhoea (or their carers) should be asked questions about the following areas:
   a. the date of onset or duration of diarrhoea stools
   b. presence of blood in stool
   c. vomiting

2 Children under 3 years presenting with acute diarrhoea (or their carers) should be asked questions about the following areas:
   a. the date of onset or duration of diarrhoea stools
   b. presence of blood in stool
   c. vomiting
   d. fever

3 Children under 16 years presenting with acute diarrhoea (or their carers) should be asked about their fluid intake

4 Children under 2 years presenting with acute diarrhoea (or their carers) should be asked about urine output

5 Children under 3 years presenting with diarrhoea should be examined with regard to general hydration status

Treatment

6 Antimicrobial agents should not be used in a child with diarrhoea unless there is a positive microbiological confirmation and the child is not improving

---

Overview of data sources used in this review

This review refers to the management of acute diarrhoea in children. In addition to references from Medline (1985–2000) and hand-searched papers, sources included Morbidity Statistics from General Practice: Fourth National Study 1991–2; data from the Public Health Laboratory Service, CDSC; the 1997 Guidelines of the European Society of Paediatric Gastroenterology and Nutrition (ESPGAN) Working Group on acute diarrhoea; and the *British National Formulary*.

References

1. McCormick A, Fleming D, Charlton J. Morbidity statistics from general practice: 4th national study 1991-92 carried out by the Royal College of General Practitioners, OPCS and Department of Health. HMSO, 1995

2. RCGP

3. Sibal A, Booth IW. Management of infectious diarrhoea in childhood. British Journal of Hospital Medicine 1997; 57(10): 484–487

4. Sandhu BK, Isolauri E, Walker-Smith JA et al. A multicentre study on behalf of the European Society of Paedric Gastroenterology and Nutrition Working Group on Acute Diarrhoea. Early feeding in childhood gastroenteritis. Journal of Pediatric Gastroenterology and Nutrition 1997; 24(5): 522–527

5. Burkhart DM. Management of acute gastroenteritis in children. American Family Physician 1999; 60(9): 2555–2563

6. Glass RI, Lew JF, Ganqarosa RE, LeBaron CW, Ho MS Estimates of morbidity and mortality rates for diarrheal diseases in American children. Journal of Pediatrics 1991; 118 (4 pt 2): S27–S33

7. Public Health Laboratory Service. Laboratory reports to the CDSC, March 1999. www.phls.co.uk/facts

8. Djuretic T, Ramsay M, Gay N, Wall P, Ryan M, Fleming D. An estimate of the proportion of diarrhoeal disease episodes seen by general practitioners attributable to rotavirus in children under 5 y of age in England and Wales. Acta Paediatrica Scandinavica Supplement 1999; 88(426): 38–41

9. Glass RI, Bresee JS, Parshar UD, Holman RC, Gentsch RR. First rotavirus vaccine licenced: is there really a need? Acta Paediatrica Scandinavica Supplement 1999; 88(426): 2–8

10. DeWitt TG. Acute diarrhea in children. Pediatrics in Review 1989; 11(1): 6–13

11. Fitzgerald JF. Management of acute diarrhea. Pediatric Infectious Disease Journal 1989; 8(8): 564–569

12. Northrup RS, Flanigan TP Gastroenteritis. Pediatrics in review 1994; 15(12): 461–472

13. World Health Organization The management and prevention of diarrhoea: practical guidelines, 3rd edn. Geneva: WHO, 1993

14. Finkelstein JA, Schwartz JS, Torrey S, Fleisher GR Common clinical features as predictors of bacterial diarrhea in infants. American Journal of Emergency Medicine 1989; 7(5): 469–473

15. Baraff LJ, Bass JW, Fleisher GR et al. Practice guideline for the management of infants and children 0 to 36 months of age with fever without source. Annals of Emergency Medicine 1993; 22(7): 1198–1210

16. Hart CR, Bain J. Child care in general practice, 3rd edn. London: Churchill Livingstone, 1989

17. Laney DW Jr, Cohen MB. Approach to the pediatric patient with diarrhea. Gastroenterology Clinics of North America 1993; 22(3) 499–516

18. Cohen MB. Etiology and mechanisms of acute infectious diarrhea in infants in the United States. Journal of Pediatrics 1991; 118 (4 pt 2): S34–S39

19. Richards L, Claeson M, Pierce NF. Management of acute diarrhea in children: lessons learned. Pediatric Infectious Disease Journal 1993; 12(1): 5–9

20. Walker-Smith JA, Sandhu BK, Isolauri E et al. Guidelines prepared by the ESPGAN Working Group on Acute Diarrhoea. Recommendations for feeding in childhood gastro-enteritis. European Society of Pediatric Gastroenterology and Nutrition. Journal of Pediatric Gastroenterology and Nutrition 1997; 24(5): 619–620

21. Nappert G, Barrios JM, Zello GA, Naylor JM. Oral hydration solution therapy in the management of children with rotavirus diarrhoea. Nitr Rev 2000; 58: 80–87

22. Santosham M, Greenough. WB III. Oral rehydration therapy: a global perspective. Journal of Pediatrics 1991; 118 (4 pt 2): S44–S51

23. Brown KH. Dietary management of acute childhood diarrhea: optimal timing of feeding and appropriate use of milks and mixed diets. Journal of Pediatrics 1991; 118(4 pt 2): S92–S98

24. Szajewska H, Hoekstra JH, Sandhu B. Management of acute gastroenteritis in Europe and the impact of the new recommendations. Journal of Pediatric Gastroenterology and Nutrition 200; 30(5): 522–527

25. Hoghton MA, Mittal NK, Sandhu BK, Mahdi G. Effects of immediate modified feeding on infantile gastro-enteritis. British Journal of General Practice 1996; 46(404): 173–175

26. Brown KH, Peerson JM, Fontaine O. Use of nonhuman milks in the dietary management of young children with acute diarrhea: a meta-analysis of clinical trials. Pediatrics 1994; 93(1): 17–27

27. British National Formulary (BNF), March. London: British Medical Association, 1999

28. Hamilton JR. Treatment of acute diarrhea. Pediatric Clinics of North America 1985; 32(2): 419–427

29. Avery ME, Snyder JD. Oral therapy for acute diarrhea: the underused simple solution. New England Journal of Medicine 1990; 323(13): 891–894

30. World Health Organization The rational use of drugs in the management of acute diarrhoea in children. Geneva: WHO, 1990
31. Ludan AC. Current management of acute diarrhoeas. Use and abuse of drug therapy. Drugs 1988; 36 (suppl 4): 18–25
32. Pickering LK. Therapy for acute infectious diarrhea in children. Journal of Pediatrics 1991; 118 (4 pt 2): S118–S128

▶12

Acute otitis media

Paul Little

Importance

Otitis media is one of the commonest infections managed in primary care, but there is great variation in diagnosis and management, with particular controversy about the role of antibiotics. Recurrent acute otitis media (AOM) is defined by some authors as 3 episodes of AOM over a 6-month period.[1,2] Recurrent AOM has a familial tendency, is more likely in those with a first episode under the age of 1 year,[2] and more likely with daycare attendance and low socio-economic status. The long-term outlook for most children with ear infections is good: adults who remember having had ear infections in childhood are no more likely to suffer hearing impairment when compared to those who do not remember suffering from ear infections.[3]

Review of evidence relating to indicator set

Diagnosis

Patients with otitis media usually experience ear pain (otalgia), fever, hearing loss,[4] and non-specific symptoms such as irritability, lethargy, decreased appetite, vomiting and diarrhoea. The non-specific symptoms are particularly common in infants.[5] Unless there is another clear source for non-specific symptoms the ear should be examined otoscopically to observe for redness, opacity, bulging drum and/or perforation in order to confirm the diagnosis, exclude mastoiditis and exclude the need for further investigation (e.g. for urinary tract infection) or admission (for septic screen) (indicator 1).

The precise diagnostic criteria for AOM differ according to national perspectives (US/Europe) and speciality (secondary/primary care).[6-13] There is little debate about the diagnosis of otitis media when florid clinical signs are present (dull drum with severe inflammation, bulging drum and/or perforation with discharge), but pneumatic otoscopy to confirm reduced mobility of the tympanic membrane has been advocated by some authorities, particularly for early presentations without florid clinical signs.[8,9] Although the reliability of pneumatic otoscopy is promising for chronic otitis media with effusion,[10] the specificity is only modest even when performed by trained health professionals.[14] A systematic review of the diagnostic accuracy of pneumatic otoscopy provides no evidence of its validity in AOM compared to microbiological/virological evidence of infection, nor its reliability in typical primary care settings.[10] Furthermore, pneumatic otoscopy is not used routinely in clinical practice in European primary care,[6,7,12,13] and few GPs have been trained in the use of pneumatic otoscopy. Finally there is concern that using the pneumatic otoscope when the drum is acutely inflamed is likely to inflict unnecessary pain on the patient. In the UK diagnosis currently and for the foreseeable future will be made on an accurate history and appearances of the tympanic membrane.[6,7] The main concern about diagnosis on clinical grounds (and where US authorities argue is the main role of the pneumatic otoscope) is for milder early cases such as children with a fever, coryza and/or who have been crying and may have a pink eardrum. In such cases, unless there is clearer evidence of significant tympanic membrane pathology, a diagnosis of otitis media should not be made.

Treatment

Antibiotic treatment

Relief of symptoms
A systematic review of controlled trials of the treatment of AOM suggest that 18 children have to be treated with antibiotics for 1 child to benefit from resolution of symptoms between 2 and 7 days after seeing the doctor[15] and that treatment doubles the risk of side-effects. A recent trial in the under 2s suggests that the symptomatic benefit is of a similar magnitude to benefit in older children.[13] The largest trial from primary care to date in 315 children aged 6 months and over compares immediate antibiotics with a delayed approach (waiting 72 hours). This trial suggests that there is little symptomatic relief from antibiotics during the first 24 hours,[16] and that the benefit from antibiotics occurs when symptoms are starting to settle anyway. The marginal advantages of immediate treatment for symptomatic relief have to be balanced against the potential disadvantages, including the medicalisation of a self-limiting illness (25% more parents will believe in the importance of antibiotics[16]), the side-effects of treatments (10% of children will get diarrhoea who would not otherwise[15,16]) and the problem of increasing antibiotic resistance.[17-22]

A systematic review found no evidence that any one class of antibiotic was superior.[23] Thus on grounds of cost-effectiveness the standard treatment should be amoxycillin, or erythromycin if the child is allergic to penicillin. A systematic review comparing short courses of treatment (5 days) with longer courses (8–10 days) showed that treatment failure, relapse or reinfection was slightly more likely with shorter courses at 8–19 days, but not significant by 20–30 days.[24] Furthermore 10-day courses with antibiotic given 3 times per day are more likely to cause diarrhoea.[25]

Prevention of major complications
The evidence from an old quasi randomised study suggests that in the past antibiotic treatment was likely to significantly reduce the incidence of acute mastoiditis from 17% in untreated groups to 0–1.5% in antibiotic-treated children.[26] However, such data are not likely to apply in healthier modern populations. A large case series from Holland in 5000 children aged 2 years and over demonstrated that a 72-hour wait-and-see policy is safe. Using this policy, antibiotics are advised for the 3% of children who

have either (1) significant otalgia and fever (>38°C) 72 hours after seeing the doctor or (2) discharge persisting for more than 14 days.[12] In this series one child had mastoiditis initially and was excluded from the wait-and-see policy. Another child developed mastoiditis, and this was a child randomised to receive myringotomy alone, and who remained unwell for 1 week (i.e. much longer than 72 hours): the child was given antibiotics and recovered. The incidence of complications of not treating (even assuming that the one case is a genuine complication) is of the same order of magnitude as anaphylaxis, the major complication of treating.[27] The wait-and-see approach with symptomatic management has also been shown to be very acceptable to parents in a trial of more than 300 children: 80% of parents will be extremely or very satisfied with this approach.[16]

There is arguably a case for treating younger children more aggressively in view of the possible greater risk of mastoiditis.[28] However, there is no good trial or cohort evidence on which to firmly guide treatment (the above report is a case series, and reporting bias is likely). The only trial to date specifically addressing those under the age of 2 years[13] showed similar estimates of efficacy to recent trials from primary care in a broader range of children.[6,15,16] Furthermore there are three contrary case reports documenting that the increasing rate of mastoiditis is related to penicillin-insensitive/resistant organisms.[29-31] This suggests that the solution to the problem of acute mastoiditis may be the *more* selective use of antibiotics for all acute infections, including AOM. It seems reasonable for younger children (under the age of 2) who are more likely to get mastoiditis, that if severe symptoms persist for more than 24 hours after seeing the doctor despite symptomatic relief then antibiotics can be used. This is in line with current Dutch practice.[32] Although most children present within 24 hours, it seems sensible to build the average preconsultation wait into the delayed prescription approach: children who have already had severe otalgia and fever for 72 hours should probably not wait and see for a further 72 hours. Thus adding 24 hours (the average time to presentation) to the 72-hour approach used in the Dutch studies gives the average total wait and see time (i.e. 96 hours total for children aged 2 and over, or 48 hours for the under 2s) (indicator 2).

There is current debate about 'otitis-prone' children – children with recurrent otitis media who have more than 2 attacks of otitis media in 6 months. Although recurrent attacks of otitis media may be a risk factor for the development of hearing impairment, it is unclear if the treatment with antibiotics for acute attacks will prevent these sequelae. However, since this group is at higher risk, and they are a small minority of children, there is at least some argument for treating these children with antibiotics more aggressively.

Non-antibiotic treatment
Non-steroidal anti-inflammatory drugs (NSAIDs) may be effective,[33,34] but have not been shown to be better than paracetamol.[35] Auralgan solution (antipyrine/benzocaine/glycerin) may also help.[36] There is no clear benefit from antihistamines or decongestants from several trials[37-42] and side-effects are more common.[37,43-45] One small trial in a specific group (acute otitis media with effusion) reported some benefit of antihistamine/decongestants.[46] Thus antihistamine/decongestants should probably

not be prescribed since at best they are likely to provide marginal benefit, and may have significant side-effects in young children (indicator 3).

Follow-up

Where perforation has occurred either at the time of presentation to the doctor, or if the child develops a discharge subsequently, children should probably be examined after 6 weeks. The purpose of this is to check healing of the tympanic membrane (ongoing perforation makes further infection and hearing impairment more likely), and if the drum is not healed children should probably be referred to an otolaryngologist.

Recommended quality indicators for acute otitis media

Diagnosis
1 Young children (under 2 years old), presenting in person to the clinician, who have systemic upset (one or more of: fever, irritability, lethargy, vomiting) with no other obvious cause should be examined including an ear examination using an otoscope

Treatment
2 Antibiotics should not be offered in children aged 2 years and over with uncomplicated acute otitis media (no ENT malformations, recurrent infections or immunocompromised), unless there is persistent fever, otalgia or discharge 72 hours after seeing the doctor (or 96 hours in total)
3 Children with acute otitis media should not be prescribed oral decongestants

---

Prevention

There is debate as to whether providing prophylaxis for otitis-prone children will reduce the incidence of infections: a meta-analysis[47] was criticised for including unusual populations (Eskimos and asthmatics) and showed a rate difference of 0.11 episodes per month comparing placebo with antibiotics (i.e. 9 children treated for 1 month to prevent 1 episode). This reduces to 0.07 when the unusual groups are excluded, and by including 4 additional trials since the review, reduces still further to 0.036, i.e. a marginal effect of treating 28 children for 1 month to prevent 1 episode.[48]

There is mixed evidence for the efficacy of pneumococcal vaccine.[49-52] Influenza A vaccination may decrease the incidence of otitis media for children aged 6–30 months in daycare.[53] Xylitol chewing gum may also help prevent recurrent otitis media,[54] but an antihistamines/decongestant mixture probably has little effect.[55]

Overview of data sources used in this review

The review is based on a search of the Cochrane Library database of systematic reviews and randomised controlled trials using the term 'otitis' and a search of

Medline 1966–1999 using the terms 'otitis media' (exploded) and 'otological diagnosis', or 'sensitivity' and 'specificity' as subject headings, or 'pneumatic' as a text word.

References

1. Teele D, Klein J, Rosner B. Epidemiology of otitis media during the first seven years of life in children in greater Boston: A prospective cohort study. Journal of Infectious Diseases 1989; 160(1): 83–94
2. Fliss D, Leiberman A, Dagan R. Medical sequelae and complications of acute otitis media. Pediatric Infectious Disease Journal 1994; 13(1): s34–s40
3. Stephenson H, Higson J, Haggard M. Binaural hearing in adults with histories of otitis media in childhood. Audiology 1995; 34: 113–123
4. Schwarz R, Rodriguez W, Brook I. The febrile response in acute otitis media. Journal of the American Medical Association 1981; 245(20): 2057–2058
5. Baker R. Pitfalls in diagnosing acute otitis media. Pediatric Annals 1991; 20(11): 591–598
6. Burke P, Bain J, Robinson D, Dunleavey J. Acute red ear in children: controlled trial of non-antibiotic treatment in general practice. British Medical Journal 1991; 303: 558–562
7. Bain J. Controversies in therapeutics. Childhood otalgia. Justification for antibiotic use in general practice. British Medical Journal 1990; 300: 1006–1007
8. Gates G, Northern J, Ferrer P et al. Diagnosis and screening. Annals of Otology and Laryngology 1989; 98 (suppl 139): 39–41
9. Schwartz R, Rodriguez W, Brook I, Grundfast K. The febrile response in otitis media. Journal of the American Medical Association 1981; 245: 2057–2058
10. Preston K. Pneumatic otoscopy: a review of the literature. Issues In Comprehensive Pediatric Nursing 1998; 21(2): 117–128
11. Ruuskanen O, Heikkinen T. Otitis media: etiology and diagnosis. Pediatric Infectious Disease Journal 1994; 13: s23–s26
12. Van Buchem FL, Peeters MF, Van 'T Hof MA. Acute otitis media a new treatment strategy. British Medical Journal 1985; 290: 1033–1037
13. Damoiseaux R, Van Balen F, Hoes A, Verheij T, De Melker R. Primary care based randomised double blind trial of amoxicillin versus placebo for acute otitis media in children aged under 2 years. British Medical Journal 2000; 320: 350–354
14. DeMelker R. Evaluation of the diagnostic value of pneumatic otoscopy in primary care using the results of tympanometry as reference standard. British Journal of General Practice 1993; 43: 22–24
15. Del Mar C, Glaziou P, Hayem M. Are antibiotics indicated as initial treatment for children with acute otitis media? A meta-analysis. British Medical Journal 1997; 314: 1526–1529
16. Little P, Gould C, Williamson I, Moore M, Warner G, Dunleavey J. A pragmatic randomised controlled trial of two prescribing strategies for acute otitis media. British Medical Journal 2001; 322: 336–342
17. House of Lords. House of Lords Select Committee on Science and Technology: 7th report. Occasional Report, 1998
18. SMAC. Standing Medical Advisory Committee (SMAC) report. The path of least resistance. Occasional Report, 1998
19. Arason V, Kristinsson K, Sigurdsson J, Stefansdottir G, Molstad S, Gudmundsson S. Do antimicrobials increase the rate of penicillin resistant pneumococci in children? Cross sectional prevalence study. British Medical Journal 1996; 313: 387–391
20. Magee J, Pritchard E. Antibiotic prescribing and antibiotic resistance in community practice: retrospective study. British Medical Journal 1999; 319: 1239–1240
21. Reacher M, Shah A, Livermore D et al. Bacteraemia and antibiotic resistance of its pathogens reported in England and Wales between 1990 and 1998: trend analysis. British Medical Journal 2000; 320: 213–216
22. Seppala H, Klaukka T, Vuopio-Varkila J. The effect of changes in the consumption of macrolide antibiotics on erythromycin resistance in group A Streptococci. New England Journal of Medicine 1997; 337: 441–446
23. Rosenfeld RM, Cipolle RJ, Uden DL, Giebink S, Canafax DM. Clinical efficacy of antimicrobial drugs for acute otitis media: meta-analysis of 5400 children from 33 randomised trials. Journal of Pediatrics 1994; 124: 355–367
24. Kozyrskj A, Hildes Ripstein E, Longstaffe S, Wincott J, Sitar S, Klassen T. Treatment of acute otitis media with a shortened course of antibiotics: a meta-analysis. Journal of the American Medical Association 1998; 279: 1736–1742

25. Hoberman A, Paradise J, Burch D, Valinski W, Hedrick J, Aronovitz G. Equivalent efficiency and reduced occurence of diarrhoea from a new formulation of amoxycillin/clavulanate potassium for treatment of acute otitis media in children. Pediatric Infectious Disease Journal 1997; 16: 463–470

26. Rudberg R. Acute otitis media: comparative therapeutic results of sulphonamide and penicillin administered in various forms. Acta Oto-laryngologica 1954; 113(suppl): 9–79

27. Hoigne R, Zoppi M, Sonntag R. Penicillins. In: Dukes MNG, ed. Meyler's side effects of drugs. Amsterdam: Elsevier, 1992: 600–622

28. Hoppe J, Koster S, Bootz F, Niethammer D. Acute mastoiditis – relevant once again. Infection 1994; 22: 178–182

29. Kudo F, Sasamura Y. Acute mastoiditis in infants: penicillin-resistant Streptococcus pneumoniae and its therapy. Nippon Jibiinkoka Gakkai Kaiho 1998; 101: 1075–1081

30. Collison P, Farver D. Acute coalescent mastoiditis caused by antibiotic resistant organisms. South Dakota Journal of Medicine 1998; 51: 379–383

31. Antonelli P, Dhanani N, Giannoni C, Kubilis P. Impact of resistant pneumococcus on the rates of acute mastoiditis. Otolaryngology – Head and Neck Surgery 1999; 121: 190–194

32. Dalhuizen J, Zwaard A, Grol R, Mokkink H. Het handelen van huisartsen volgens de standaard Otitis media acuta van het Nederlands Huisarten Genootschap. Nederlands Tijdschrift voor Geneeskunde 1993; 137: 2139–2144

33. Schachtel B, Thoden W. Assaying analgesic response in children: a double blind placebo controlled model involving earache. Pediatric Research 1991; 29: 124a

34. Pretto G, Oliani C, Cimino G, Esposito G. Morniflumato efficacy and tolerability in the treatment of acute and subacute otitis media catarrhalis. Riv.Ital.otorinlaryngol.Audiol.Foniatr. 1991; 11: 72–77

35. Bertin L, Pons G, d'Athis P, Duhamel J, Mandelonde C, Lasfargues G. A randomised double blind multicentre controlled trial of ibuprofen versus acetaminophen and placebo for symptoms of acute otitis media in children. Fundamental and Clinical Pharmacology 1996; 10: 387–392

36. Hoberman A, Paradise J, Reynolds E, Urkin J. Efficacy of auralgan for treating ear pain in children with acute otitis media. Archives of Pediatrics and Adolescent Medicine 1997; 151: 675–678

37. Bain DJ. Can the clinical course of acute otitis media be modified by systemic decongestant-antihistamine combination for otitis media in children. British Medical Journal 1983; 287: 654–656

38. Bhambhani K, Foulds D, Swamy K, Eldis F, Fischel J. Acute otitis media in children: are decongestants or antihistamines necessary. Annals of Emergency Medicine 1983; 12: 13–16

39. Sorri M, Sipila P, Palva A, Karma P. Can secretory otitis media be prevented by oral decongestants? Acta Oto-laryngologica 1982; 94: 115–116

40. Chilton L, Skipper B. Antihistamines and alpha-adrenergic agents in the treatment of otitis media. Southern Medical Journal 1979; 72: 953–955

41. Thomsen J, Mygind N, Meistrup-Larsen K, Sorensen H, Vesterhauge S. Oral decongestants in acute otitis media. Results of a double blind study. International Journal of Pediatric Otorhinolaryngology 1979; 1: 103–108

42. Schnore S, Sangster J, Gerace T, Bass M. Are antihistamine-decongestants of value in the treatment of acute otitis media in children? Journal of Family Practice 1986; 22: 39–43

43. Cantekin E, Mandell E, Bluestone C et al. Lack of efficacy of a decongestant-antihistamine combination for otitis media with effusion ('secretory' otitis media) in children. New England Journal of Medicine 1983; 308: 297–301

44. Lewith G, Davidson F. Dystonic reactions to Dimotapp elixir. Journal of the Royal College of General Practitioners 1981; 31: 241

45. Sankey R, Nunn A, Sills J. Visual hallucinations in children receiving decongestants. British Medical Journal 1984; 288: 1369

46. Moran D, Mutchie K, Higbee M, Paul L. The use of an antihistamine decongestant in conjunction with an anti-infective drug in the treatment of acute otitis media. Journal of Pediatrics 1982; 101: 132–136

47. Williams R, Chalmers T, Strange K, Chalmers F, Bowin S. Use of antibiotics in preventing recurrent acute otitis media and in treating otitis media with effusion: a meta-analytic attempt to resolve the brouhaha. Journal of the American Medical Association 1993; 270: 1344–1351

48. Cantekin E. Where is the evidence? Electronic response to O'Neill volume. British Medical Journal 1999; 319: 833–835

49. Makela P, Leinone M, Pukander J, Karma P. A study of the pneumococcal vaccine in the prevention of clinically acute attacks of recurrent otitis media. Reviews of Infectious Diseases 1981; 3(suppl): s124–s132

50. Teele D, Klein J, Bratton L et al. Use of pneumococcal vaccine for the prevention of recurrent acute otitis media in infants in Boston. The Greater Boston Collaborative Otitis Media Study Group. Reviews of Infectious Diseases 1981; 3(suppl): s113–s118

51.   Sloyer J, Ploussard J, Howie V. Efficacy of pneumococcal polysaccharide vaccine in preventing acute otitis media in infants in Huntsville, Alabama. Reviews of Infectious Diseases 1981; 3 (suppl): s119–s123
52.   Douglas R, Miles H. Vaccination against streptococcus pneumoniae in childhood: lack of demonstrable benefit in young Australian children. Journal of Infectious Diseases 1984; 149: 861–869
53.   Clements D, Langdon L, Bland C, Walter E. Influenza A vaccine decreases the incidence of otitis media in 6–30 month old children in day care. Archives of Pediatrics and Adolescent Medicine 1995; 149: 1113–1117
54.   Uhari M, Kontiokari T, Koskelika M, Neimela M. Xylitol chewing gum in the prevention of acute otitis media: a double blind randomised trial. British Medical Journal 1996; 313: 1180–1184
55.   Randall J, Henley J. A decongestant-antihistamine mixture in the prevention of otitis media in children with colds. Pediatrics 1979; 63: 483–485

►13

Allergic rhinitis

Helen Smith and Stephen Morgan

Importance

Rhinitis is the inflammation of the mucous membrane of the nose. The condition may be seasonal or perennial. Some cases of perennial rhinitis will also show seasonal exacerbations. Most cases of seasonal rhinitis are due to allergies to airborne pollens. About half of the cases of perennial rhinitis are allergic in origin, the remainder being due to vasomotor instability, or part of a more extensive rhinosinusitis.

Although allergic rhinitis and hayfever affect 10–20% of the population, only a minority consult their GP.[1-3] Many sufferers self-medicate with treatments available without prescription and often have trivial symptoms. Although rarely causing life-threatening complications, the restriction of normal activities and the loss of time from school or work have substantial impact on quality of life.

Review of evidence relating to quality indicators

Diagnosis

Patient history is the key diagnostic tool in allergic rhinitis. Symptoms include nasal congestion, rhinorrhoea, sneezing, and itching of the nasopharynx and eyes.[4,5] The history may enable symptoms to be related to specific allergens. The pattern of use of medications, including topical nasal preparation, should be identified.

Examination of the nasal mucosa using an auroscope may reveal pale, swollen nasal turbinates and clear secretions. Fever, purulent rhinorrhoea and enlarged cervical lymph nodes make the diagnosis of an infective upper airway condition more likely.[6]

Skin prick testing by suitably trained staff using standardised allergens and protocols can be useful to confirm specific allergen sensitivity but there is a significant proportion (approximately 15%) of false-positive results, i.e. patients with positive skin tests whose rhinitis is non-allergic in origin. Testing therefore needs careful interpretation.[6,7]

Treatment

Treatment options include allergen avoidance, use of drugs and specific immunotherapy. Allergen avoidance advice should be considered in all cases but needs to be tailored to the level of symptoms, the effectiveness of alternative treatments and the impact of avoidance measures on quality of life.[8]

First-line drug treatments include oral antihistamines with second-generation agents generally preferred unless sedative side-effects are either desirable or insignificant. Antihistamines have relatively little effect on nasal blockage and if this is a prominent symptom greater benefit is likely if a nasal corticosteroid is used as an alternative or additional treatment.[9] Nasal corticosteroids do not have any effect on eye symptoms. For maximal effect they need to be taken on a regular basis and, where possible, commenced before the beginning of the symptomatic season.[6] Nasal sodium cromoglycate is an alternative but requires regular 4 times daily treatment to be effective.

Systemic corticosteroids have a relatively high potential for serious side-effects and thus should only be used in short-term treatment of urgent or severe cases alongside optimised first-line therapies. In these unusual circumstances, oral rather than parenteral treatment should be used[10] (indicator 2).

Oral and topical decongestants (α agonists) can be used with the other therapies in line with their published indications. Topical decongestant therapy should be limited to a maximum of 1 week (indicator 1). There is some evidence to support the use of topical nasal ipratropium bromide or topical antihistamines (H_1 antagonist). Oral ketotifen or H_2 antagonist have also been used in trials but these are not recommended as first-line agents.[6]

Specific immunotherapy can be considered where optimal alternative treatments have been ineffective and the symptoms are persistent and disabling.[11] As specific immunotherapy can have serious adverse effects it should be conducted under the supervision of an allergy specialist with suitable resuscitation equipment available. It is not suitable for patients with uncontrolled asthma.[7]

Recommended quality indicators for acute allergic rhinitis

Treatment
1 If nasal decongestants are prescribed for patients with allergic rhinitis, then they should not be prescribed for longer than 1 week in any 3-month period
2 If systemic corticosteroids are prescribed they should:
   a. not be for longer than 14 days
   b. not be by injection
   c. only be prescribed after an adequate course of antihistamines and topical treatment have proven to be ineffective or were not tolerated

---

Overview of data sources used in this review

This review is based on review articles cited in Medline and Embase (from January 1996 to October 1999), the Cochrane Library of systematic reviews, the Database of Abstracts of Reviews of Effectiveness, the Drug and Therapeutics Bulletin, the MeReC Bulletin, consensus reports from the International Rhinitis Management Working Group, the UK Royal Colleges of Physicians alone and in conjunction with the Royal College of Pathologists and the British Society for Allergy and Clinical Immunology. Local experts were also consulted.

Further reading

British Society for Allergy and Clinical Immunology ENT Subcommittee. Rhinitis management guidelines. London: Martin Dunitz, 2000

Durham SR, ed. ABC of allergies. London: BMA, 1998

Scadding GK, Mygind N. Fast facts; allergic rhinitis. Oxford: Health Press, 2000

References

1. Jones NS, Smith PA, Carney AS, Davis A. The prevalence of allergic rhinitis and nasal symptoms in Nottingham. Clinical Otolaryngology and Allied Sciences 1998; 23: 547–554
2. Austin JB, Kaur B, Anderson HR et al. Hay fever, eczema, and wheeze: a nationwide UK study (ISAAC, international study of asthma and allergies in childhood). Archives of Disease in Childhood 1999; 81: 225–230
3. Sibbald B, Rink E. Epidemiology of seasonal and perennial rhinitis: clinical presentation and medical history. Thorax 1991; 46: 895–901
4. Rhinitis: consensus statement. 2nd edn. London: British Society of Allergy and Clinical Immunology, 1996
5. Parikh A, Scadding GK. Seasonal allergic rhinitis. British Medical Journal 1997; 314: 1392–1395
6. Anonymous. International consensus report on the diagnosis and management of rhinitis. International Rhinitis Management Working Group. Allergy 1994; 49: 1–34
7. Anonymous. Good allergy practice – standards of care for providers and purchasers of allergy services within the National Health Service. Royal College of Physicians and Royal College of Pathologists. Clinical and Experimental Allergy 1995; 25: 586–595
8. Naclerio RM. Allergic rhinitis. New England Journal of Medicine 1991; 325: 860–869
9. Durham S. ABC of allergies. Summer hay fever. British Medical Journal 1998; 316: 843–845
10. Anonymous. Any place for triamcinolone in hay fever? Drug and Therapeutics Bulletin 1999; 37: 17–18
11. Malling HJ. Immunotherapy as an effective tool in allergy treatment. Allergy 1998; 53: 461–472

14

Dyspepsia and peptic ulcer disease

Brendan Delaney

Uninvestigated dyspepsia: importance

Expenditure on ulcer-healing drugs is the highest cost therapeutic group, at an annual cost to the NHS in excess of £500 million. Dyspepsia is common, with an incidence of 2 per 1000 population per year, but dyspepsia is also a lifelong intermittent and relapsing disorder.[1] Studies have shown that as many as 3% of the population may be taking long-term prescribed medication for dyspepsia.[2] In any 6-month period 40% of the population will suffer an episode of dyspepsia, and half of those will consult their general practitioner.[3]

Review of evidence relating to quality indicators for uninvestigated dyspepsia

Screening

Only 1 in 4 of all patients with dyspepsia consult their general practitioner.[4] As there is no good evidence that early intervention for dyspepsia is more effective than current practice, routine screening of individuals for dyspepsia is not indicated.

Diagnosis

Symptom patterns are not sensitive or specific enough to make a diagnosis of the underlying cause of dyspepsia.[5,6] Patients with predominant reflux symptoms (heartburn, acid regurgitation) may have gastro-oesophageal reflux disease (GORD). Although symptoms are not specific for *oesophagitis*, reflux symptoms often respond well to acid suppression, particularly with a proton pump inhibitor (PPI), and the response of heartburn symptoms to a PPI has been used to substantiate a diagnosis of GORD. Patients with recurrent dyspepsia and a previous peptic ulcer may have recurrent peptic ulcer disease, so this diagnosis should be clearly recorded in the patient notes (indicator 1).

Use of current medications should be determined in patients with dyspepsia. Aspirin or non-steroidal anti-inflammatory drugs (NSAIDs) are particularly important, as these may cause gastritis or ulcers[7-11] (indicator 2). The 2–4% overall risk of ulcers in patients taking NSAIDs is twice that of the general population,[12] and 4–5 times higher than that of age-matched controls in elderly people.[7,8] Drug-induced dyspepsia may also occur with corticosteroids,[13] theophylline, digoxin, oral antibiotics (especially ampicillin and erythromycin), or potassium or iron supplements.[14]

Patients over the age of 55 years with recent onset of symptoms or constant pain and all those patients with symptoms suggestive of malignancy (weight loss, dysphagia, early satiety, jaundice or anaemia) should be investigated by prompt endoscopy[15,16] (indicator 3).

Treatment

A number of strategies for managing dyspeptic patients incorporating non-invasive tests for *Helicobacter pylori* followed by either endoscopy or *H. pylori* eradication therapy restricted to those testing positive have been suggested.

Empirical antisecretory therapy/treat and endoscope

This involves treating dyspeptic patients with antacids, H_2 receptor antagonists or PPIs and only investigating those that fail to respond. This strategy reserves costly investigation to those patients who are consuming more medication, hence the cost of investigation might be recovered by decreased prescribing. However, patients with peptic ulcer disease may receive intermittent antisecretory drugs, responding promptly at each recurrence, whereas *H. pylori* eradication is now the treatment of choice for this group.[17] Nevertheless empirical antisecretory therapy or early endoscopy is the usual approach taken by general practitioners when initially investigating younger patients with dyspepsia.

Early endoscopy

An alternative strategy is to investigate all dyspeptic patients before initiating a prescription. This strategy takes into account the potential for patients over the age of 50 to have underlying upper gastrointestinal cancer. Approximately 1 in 300 patients had a potentially curable gastric cancer in a large cohort study of unrestricted early endoscopy in Birmingham.[18] Sufficiently large randomised controlled trials are unlikely to be carried out and cost-effectiveness is likely to be low. A meta-analysis of 3 prospective randomised studies[19-21] has indicated that early endoscopy as a strategy may be more effective in terms of cure of dyspeptic symptoms than empirical antacid therapy, particularly in the older age group. Incorporation of a further large trial gives a relative risk of 0.88 (95% CI 0.77–1.00) for dyspepsia in initial endoscopy compared with usual management.[22]

Initial endoscopy is associated with additional costs. The economic analysis from one of these studies has been published, indicating that the incremental cost-effectiveness ratio of initial endoscopy compared with usual management is £1728 per patient free of symptoms at a baseline cost of endoscopy of £246. A sensitivity analysis showed that if the cost of endoscopy could fall to £100 the incremental cost-effectiveness ratio would fall to only £165.[23]

Non-invasive H. pylori testing and endoscopy

H. pylori may be identified by urea breath testing (UBT), serology, stool antigen tests or near patient tests (NPT). UBT and stool antigens are more accurate, but more costly than serology or NPTs. At present there is insufficient evidence as to which test is most cost-effective for initial diagnosis in primary care, but serology or NPT cannot be used as a predictor of cure (indicator 4).

Strategies based on testing for *H. pylori* have been proposed. These include selective endoscopy only in those patients testing positive (test and scope)[24] and *H. pylori* eradication.[25,26] *H. pylori* is associated with nearly all peptic ulcers in patients not taking NSAIDs. A strategy of screening patients for *H. pylori* with serology or UBT and only investigating those infected has been suggested by several groups. This could reduce endoscopies in young dyspeptics by 23–66% while detecting almost 100% of peptic ulcers in those not taking NSAIDs.[27] A recent primary care-based randomised controlled trial has shown that test and scope is more costly than usual management in primary care, and does not lead to any difference in dyspeptic symptoms.[28]

Non-invasive H. pylori *testing and eradication*
Two trials where patients were randomised after testing to either *H. pylori* eradication or PPI/placebo have been completed, but neither is yet published in full. The Cadet-HP study, set in primary care in Canada, showed a significant reduction in recurrent dyspeptic symptoms from 54% to 40% with eradication versus PPI alone at 1 year.[29] A similar trial in Finland found that the period prevalence of peptic ulcer disease was reduced from 6.2% to 1% during the 2 years after eradication therapy, compared with placebo.[30]

Several trials comparing test and eradicate with endoscopy in secondary care have been conducted. Heaney found that *H. pylori* eradication was more effective than endoscopy in reducing dyspeptic symptoms in patients under the age of 45 years. At 1 year of follow-up 57% of the 'test-and-treat' group had dyspepsia compared with 70% of the endoscopy group (RR 0.81, 95% CI 0.51–1.19).[31] Lassen[32] randomised 500 patients referred by general practitioners with uninvestigated dyspepsia to test-and-treat or endoscopy. Symptoms were similar at 1 year, but the use of endoscopy in the test-and-treat group was 60% less than in the endoscopy group.[32]

Medication

Antacids
Antacids are safe, cheap and effective drugs. The main disadvantage is the frequency with which they need to be taken, up to 7 times a day.

H_2 receptor antagonists
H_2 receptor antagonists are potent inhibitors of acid secretion, but less effective than PPIs. An inconclusive single randomised controlled trial has compared H_2 receptor antagonists with antacids in primary care.[33] Evidence is lacking as to their relative cost-effectiveness.

Proton pump inhibitors
A systematic review has found that, in the short-term, PPIs were more effective at controlling dyspeptic symptoms in unselected patients in primary care than both

antacids and H_2 receptor antagonists. Pooled relative risks were 0.71 (0.64–0.79) for PPI versus antacids and 0.63 (0.47–0.85) for PPI versus H_2 receptor antagonists. The effect on heartburn was greater (RR 0.52, 0.45–0.60), but epigastric pain did not respond as well, in fact for this there was no significant difference between PPI and antacids for epigastric pain.[22]

Prokinetics
There is insufficient evidence to determine the effectiveness of prokinetic agents in unselected dyspeptic patients in primary care. Cisapride has recently had its UK licence suspended.

H. pylori *eradication*
The simplest *H. pylori* management strategy of all would be to prescribe empirical *H. pylori* eradication therapy to all young dyspeptic patients. This avoids the inconvenience and cost of testing for *H. pylori* and a published model[12] has suggested that this may be the most cost-effective strategy for managing dyspepsia. Empirical treatment was only slightly cheaper than the screening and treatment strategy and resulted in 50–70% of young dyspeptics who are *H. pylori* negative receiving antibiotics unnecessarily. Whether the increase in antibiotic exposure is worth this small cost saving is debatable, and given current concerns over antibiotic resistance, empirical eradication is not recommended.

Follow-up

Follow-up for dyspepsia is a concern only if complicated peptic ulcer disease is identified. Management and follow-up for peptic ulcer disease are discussed below.

Peptic ulcer disease: importance

Peptic ulcer disease is found in less than 10% of patients undergoing endoscopy for dyspepsia. The Fourth National Morbidity Survey in General Practice found consultation rates of 0.5% per year and new episode rates of 0.4% per year for peptic ulcer disease.[1] Peptic ulcer disease is the leading cause of acute haemorrhage of the upper gastrointestinal tract, accounting for about 50% of all cases. Despite advances in treatment, overall mortality has remained at approximately 6–8% for the past 30 years, due in part to increasing patient age and prevalence of concurrent illness.[34]

Review of evidence relating to indicators for peptic ulcer disease

Screening

Modelling studies have suggested that screening for and eradicating *H. pylori* in asymptomatic patients may be a cost-effective approach to reducing both the incidence of peptic ulcer disease and distal gastric cancer.[35] Until evidence from ongoing trials is available, treating asymptomatic patients who have *H. pylori* for primary prevention of ulcers is not recommended.

Prevention

Use of NSAIDs

Misoprostol, PPIs and H_2 blockers have been used to prevent NSAID-induced ulcers. Specific cyclo-oxygenase-2 inhibitors are now available. As yet, there are insufficient data from primary care to indicate the cost-effectiveness of these agents.

Diagnosis

Endoscopy

Peptic ulcers are detected by the presence of a distinct crater that is visible on radiological or endoscopic examination of the upper gastrointestinal tract; they differ from erosions in that ulcers penetrate beyond the mucosa to the submucosa.[9] Modelling suggests that patients with a previous history of peptic ulcer, who are still infected with *H. pylori*, are likely to have a recurrent ulcer if they become symptomatic again.[36] Further endoscopy is probably not necessary in such patients, who should receive eradication therapy.

Testing for H. pylori *in peptic ulcer disease*

Several tests are available for evaluating infection with *H. pylori*. Serological testing is sensitive and specific, and is the least expensive method. However, because serological testing does not distinguish between past and current *H. pylori* infection, it cannot be used to test for recurrence or for effect of treatment. Gastric mucosal biopsy – by staining of biopsy materials, the *Campylobacter*-like organism test, or *H. pylori* culture – and the C_{13}-UBT may be used repeatedly to check for eradication of *H. pylori*. *H. pylori* produces urease that hydrolyses labelled urea, producing NH_3 and $^{13}CO_2$; $^{13}CO_2$ is identified in expired air by mass spectroscopy. Culture is the least sensitive of the direct techniques.

The UBT has the advantage of being non-invasive. These latter methods are sensitive to bacterial load and should be performed at least 4 weeks after use of bismuth or eradication therapy, because recent *H. pylori* suppression without eradication can lead to false-negative results. [37]

Treatment

Uncomplicated peptic ulcer disease

Management of uncomplicated peptic ulcer disease centres around the eradication of *H. pylori*.[35] All patients with peptic ulcer disease, either newly diagnosed or a prior diagnosis, should receive *H. pylori* eradication therapy. Eradication of *H. pylori*, if it is present, and avoidance of NSAIDs have been proven to cure more than 95% of patients with peptic ulcer disease[38] (indicator 5). A meta-analysis has shown that 1-week PPI-based triple therapies can achieve more than 80% cure in intention-to-treat analysis of trials and are well tolerated[39] (indicator 6).

Complicated peptic ulcer disease

Complicated peptic ulcer disease is defined as peptic ulcer disease associated with bleeding, perforation or obstruction. Gastrointestinal bleeding is the most common of these complications. Patients with suspected gastrointestinal bleeding should be referred as an emergency to secondary care.

Follow-up

Confirmation of H. pylori eradication

Confirmation of successful *H. pylori* cure by endoscopic biopsy or UBT is important in patients with a history of ulcers complicated by bleeding, perforation, or obstruction, or ulcers that recur after *H. pylori* eradication therapy.[40] Successful eradication of *H. pylori* has been clearly shown to reduce bleeding recurrences, while *H. pylori* persistence after therapy is associated with continued risk of rebleeding.[41] Confirmation of eradication is not necessary in patients with uncomplicated ulcers who remain asymptomatic after antibiotic therapy.[37] Eradication therapy has been shown to reduce duodenal ulcer recurrences at 1 year from 80% to 5%.[42]

Recommended quality indicators for dyspepsia

Diagnosis
1 The diagnosis of peptic ulcer disease should be clearly identifiable on the electronic or paper records
2 For patients consulting with dyspepsia enquiry should be made about:
   a. previous history of peptic ulcer disease
   b. use of NSAIDs
   c. presence or absence of 'alarm symptoms' (weight loss, early satiety, dysphagia, haematemesis, melaena)

Investigation
3 Patients with alarm symptoms (weight loss, early satiety, dysphagia, haematemesis, melaena) should be referred for urgent endoscopy or specialist referral at first presentation to the GP
4 *H. pylori* serology should be for initial diagnosis only, not as a test for cure

Treatment
5 *H. pylori* eradication should be offered to patients with proven duodenal ulcer disease (confirmatory test not necessary) with active symptoms and who have not had H. Pylorieradiation previously
6 *H. pylori* eradication regime should consist of a PPI + 2 antibiotics for a week

---

Overview of data sources used in this review

This review is based on a recent systematic review funded by the NHS R&D HTA programme.[43] The Cochrane Collaboration Controlled Trials Register, The Cochrane Collaboration Database of Systematic Reviews, Medline, EMBASE, CINAHL, SIGLE (System for Information on the Grey Literature in Europe), Integrated Sciences Citation Index (ISCI via the Bath Information and Data Services–BIDS) were searched up until January 1999. Experts in the field of dyspepsia, major pharmaceutical companies, and journal editors were also contacted. Authors of publications in abstract only were contacted for the full trial results.

References

1. McCormick A, Fleming D, Charlton J. Morbidity statistics from general practice. Fourth national morbidity study 1991–1992. London: Office of Population Censuses and Surveys, 1995
2. Ryder SD, O'Reilly S, Miller RJ, Ross J, Jacyna MR, Levi AJ. Long term acid suppressing treatment in general practice. British Medical Journal 1994; 308(6932): 827–830
3. Jones RH, Lydeard S. Prevalence of symptoms of dyspepsia in the community. British Medical Journal 1989; 298(6665): 30–32
4. Jones RH. Dyspeptic symptoms in the community. Gut 1989; 30(7): 893–898
5. Talley NJ, Weaver AL, Tesmer DL, Zinsmeister AR. Lack of discriminant value of dyspepsia subgroups in patients referred for upper endoscopy. Gastroenterology 1993; 105(5): 1378–1386
6. Bytzer P, Hansen JM, Havelund T, Malchow-Moller A, Schaffalitzky de Muckadell OB. Predicting endoscopic diagnosis in the dyspeptic patient: the value of clinical judgement. European Journal of Gastroenterology and Hepatology 1996; 8(4): 359–363
7. Griffin MR, Piper JM, Daugherty JR, Snowden M, Ray WA. Nonsteroidal anti-inflammatory drug use and increased risk for peptic ulcer disease in elderly persons. Annals of Internal Medicine 1991; 114(4): 257–263
8. Griffin MR, Ray WA, Schaffner W. Nonsteroidal anti-inflammatory drug use and death from peptic ulcer in elderly persons. Annals of Internal Medicine 1988; 109(5): 359–363
9. Clearfield HR. Management of NSAID-induced ulcer disease (review, 12 refs). American Family Physician 1992; 45(1): 255–258
10. Smith PM, Troughton AH, Gleeson F, Walters J, McCarthy CF. Pirenzepine in non-ulcer dyspepsia: a double-blind multicentre trial. Journal of International Medical Research 1990; 18(1): 16–20
11. Lee J, O'Morain C. Who should be treated for Helicobacter pylori infection? A review of consensus conferences and guidelines. Gastroenterology 1997; 113(6 suppl): S99–S106
12. Ebell MH, Warbasse L, Brenner C. Evaluation of the dyspeptic patient: a cost-utility study. Journal of Family Practice 1997; 44(6): 545–555
13. DePriest JL. Stress ulcer prophylaxis. Do critically ill patients need it? (Review, 23 refs). Postgraduate Medicine 1996; 98(4): 159–161. Published erratum, Postgraduate Medicine 1997; 101(1): 36
14. Pound SE, Heading RC. Diagnosis and treatment of dyspepsia in the elderly. Drugs and Aging 1995; 7: 347–354
15. Axon ATR, Bell GD, Jones RH, Quine MA, McCloy RF. Guidelines on appropriate indications for upper gastrointestinal endoscopy. British Medical Journal 1995; 310: 853–856
16. Anonymous. Referral guidelines for suspected cancer. London. NHS Executive, 2000
17. Agreus L, Talley NJ. Dyspepsia: current understanding and management. Annual Review of Medicine 1998; 49: 475–493
18. Hallissey MT, Allum WH, Jewkes AJ, Ellis DJ, Fielding JW. Early detection of gastric cancer. British Medical Journal 1990; 301(6751): 513–515
19. Delaney BC, Wilson S, Roalfe A, Roberts L, Redman V, Weam AM, Briggs A, Hobbs FDR. Cost-effectiveness of inital endoscopy for dyspepsia in patients over the age of 50 years: A randomised controlled trial in primary care. Lancet 2000; 356: 1965–1969
20. Lewin-van den Broek NT. Diagnostic and therapeutic strategies for dyspepsia in primary care. Utrecht: Thesis Universitiet Utrecht, 1999
21. de Groot GH, de Both PS. Cisapride in functional dyspepsia in general practice. A placebo-controlled, randomized, double-blind study. Alimentary Pharmacology and Therapeutics 1997; 11(1): 193–199
22. Delaney BC, Innes MA, Deeks J et al. Initial management strategies for dyspepsia (full Cochrane review) (computer program). 2. Oxford: Update Software, 2000
23. Wilson S, Delaney BC, Roalfe A, Redman V, Roberts L, Hobbs FDR, A primary care-based RCT of early endoscopy for dyspepsia in patients of 50 years of age and over. Endoscopy 1999; 31: E14
24. Patel P, Khulusi S, Mendall MA, Lloyd R, Jazrawi R, Maxwell JD, Northfield TC. Prospective screening of dyspeptic patients by Helicobacter pylori serology. Lancet 1995; 346(8986): 1315–1318
25. Boyd EJ, Peden NR, Browning MC, Saunders JH, Wormsley KG. Clinical and endocrine aspects of treatment with ranitidine. Scandinavian Journal of Gastroenterology 1981; 69 (suppl): 81–83
26. Jones R, Crouch SL. Low-dose lansoprazole provides greater relief of heartburn and epigastric pain than low-dose omeprazole in patients with acid-related dyspepsia. Alimentary Pharmacology and Therapeutics 1999; 13(3): 413–419

27. Sobala GM, Crabtree JE, Pentith JA et al. Screening dyspepsia by serology to Helicobacter pylori. Lancet 1991; 338(8759): 94–96

28. Delaney BC, Wilson S, Roalfe A, Roberts L, Redman V, Wearn A, Hobbs FDR, Randomised controlled trial of melicobacter pylori testing and endoscopy for dyspepsia in primary care. British Medical Journal 2001; 322

29. Chiba N, Veldhuyzen van Zanten SJ, Sinclair P et al. Beneficial effect of H. pylori eradication therapy on long term symptom relief in primary care patients with uninvestigated dyspepsia: the Cadet-HP study. (abstr) Gastroenterology 2000; 118(S4): A438

30. Farkkila MA, Sarna S, Sipponen P. 'Test-and-treat'-strategy for management of uninvestigated dyspepsia in primary healthcare. (abstr) Gastroenterology 2000; 118(S4): A438

31. Heaney A, Collins JSA, Watson RGP, McFarland RJ, Bamford KB, Tham TCK. A prospective randomised trial of a 'test and treat' policy versus endoscopy based management in young Helicobacter pylori positive patients with ulcer-like dyspepsia, referred to a hospital clinic. Gut 1999; 45: 186–190

32. Lassen AT, Pedersen FM, Bytzer P, Scaffalitzky de Muckadell OB. Helicobacter pylori 'test and eradicate' or prompt endoscopy for management of dyspeptic patients. A randomised controlled trial with one year follow-up Lancet 2000; 356: 455–460

33. Paton S. Cost-effective treatment of gastro-oesophageal reflux disease – a comparison of two therapies commonly used in general practice. British Journal of Medical Economics 1995; 8(2): 85–95

34. Laine L, Peterson WL. Bleeding peptic ulcer. New England Journal of Medicine 1994; 331(11): 717–727

35. Parsonnet J, Harris RA, Hack HM, Owens DK. Modelling cost-effectiveness of Helicobacter pylori screening to prevent gastric cancer: a mandate for clinical trials (see comments). Lancet 1996; 348(9021): 150–154

36. Briggs AH, Sculpher MJ, Logan RP, Aldous J, Ramsay ME, Baron JH. Cost effectiveness of screening for and eradication of Helicobacter pylori in management of dyspeptic patients under 45 years of age. British Medical Journal 1996; 312(7042): 1321–1325

37. Agreus L, Talley N. Challenges in managing dyspepsia in general practice. British Medical Journal 1997; 315(7118): 1284–1288

38. Jiranek GC, Kozarek RA. A cost-effective approach to the patient with peptic ulcer bleeding. Surgical Clinics of North America 1996; 76(1): 83–103

39. Unge P. What other regimens are under investigation to treat Helicobacter pylori infection? Gastroenterology 1997; 113(6 suppl): S131–S148

40. Fullerton S, Ofman JJ, Soll AH. Empiric antibiotic-therapy vs early endoscopy in dyspeptic patients with positive serologic test for helicobacter-pylori – a decision-analysis. Gastroenterology 1995; 108: A15

41. Labenz J, Borsch G. Role of Helicobacter pylori eradication in the prevention of peptic ulcer bleeding relapse. Digestion 1994; 55(1): 19–23

42. Hopkins RJ, Girardi LS, Turney EA. Relationship between Helicobacter pylori eradication and reduced duodenal and gastric ulcer recurrence: a review. Gastroenterology 1996; 110(4): 1244–1252

43. Talley NJ, Colin-Jones D, Koch KL, Koch M, Nyren O, Stanghellini V. Functional dyspepsia: a classification with guidelines for diagnosis and management. Gastroenterology International 1991; 4(4): 145–160

▶15

Headache

Norma O'Flynn and Leone Ridsdale

Importance

Headache has a high incidence and prevalence in the community, with associated morbidity. The prevalence of migraine in the last year was 6% of males and 15% of females in a Danish epidemiological study where a random sample of 25 to 64-year-olds was examined by neurologists.[1] These prevalence figures are consistent with other population studies using the International Headache Society (IHS) criteria.[2,3] The prevalence of tension headache in the last year in the Danish study was 63% among males and 86% among females.[4] Daily or near-daily headache affects almost 5% of unselected populations,[5,6] of which half is chronic tension-type headache.

Headache is commonly presented in primary care. The Fourth National Morbidity Study found a consultation rate for migraine of 115/10 000 person years at risk;[7] an incidence study in a British general practice population where new cases over 1 year were noted found an incidence of 210/100 000 for new headache and 64/100 000 for new migraine.[8]

Review of evidence relating to quality indicators

Diagnosis

Headaches are largely diagnosed as clinical syndromes. Primary headaches are those for which there is no structural or metabolic cause. The objective of the diagnostic process is to rule out secondary causes, particularly serious causes of headache, and then to accurately diagnose primary headache to ensure appropriate treatment.

History

The most common primary headaches are tension headache and migraine. Secondary headache is most commonly associated with excess alcohol consumption, medication misuse, fever and disorders of the nose and sinuses.[3] Headache type is diagnosed by focusing on the exact definition of the prominent symptoms, in particular the temporal pattern, the description of pain and associated signs and symptoms, as well as related phenomena. Primary headaches can coexist: a patient may have tension headache and migraine.

The headache history should include whether this is new-onset headache or part of a longer headache history and if so, the age of onset of headache. Characteristics of the headache itself need to be assessed, such as the location (migraine is usually unilateral but 30–40% can be bilateral), the quality (e.g. pulsating, pressure), the intensity/severity and any aggravation by movement. Prodromal features or aura are clinical features of classical migraine. Nausea or vomiting during an attack, and sensitivity to light and sound predominantly occur with migraine. Other features of headache history include family history, precipitating, exacerbating or palliating factors and a drug history.

Aspects of the history that may indicate underlying pathology are new-onset headache, particularly in middle age or later, worst-ever headache, changes in frequency or severity of usual features of previous long-standing headache, and the presence of systemic features such as fever, anorexia, weight loss, muscle ache or jaw claudication.[9]

There is very little literature on the sensitivity and specificity of aspects of the history. In a Danish population, a questionnaire validated against a telephone interview found that the two questions 'Have you ever had migraine?' and 'Have you ever had visual disturbances lasting 5–60 min followed by headache?' identified 93% of migraineurs with aura and 75% of migraineurs without aura.[10] The findings are likely to differ in populations with less knowledge of migraine. Jaw claudication is strongly suggestive of giant cell arteritis; the odds of a positive biopsy are 9 times greater if jaw claudication is present.[11] Individual items of the clinical history have low accuracy for the diagnosis of meningitis in adults. Results from a review of studies of patients with meningitis indicated sensitivity of 50% for headache (CI 32–68%) and sensitivity of 30% for nausea/vomiting (CI 22–38%).[12]

There is evidence of comorbidity of headache and mood disorders.[13–17] These areas may need to be covered in the history.

Examination

There is lack of agreement about the essential elements of the physical examination. If the main symptom is headache, and the history has not revealed any focal symptoms, complete physical and neurological examination is not usually helpful.[18] Examinations suggested by neurologists include blood pressure and extracranial structures such as sinuses, scalp arteries, cervical paraspinal muscles and temporomandibular joints (TMJs). Suggested neurological examination includes optic fundi, cranial nerves (in particular the Vth cranial nerve, including the corneal reflex); muscle power, gait, reflexes and plantar responses. The prime objective of the examination is to support the diagnostic hypothesis suggested by the history and to exclude causes of headache that require further investigation.

There is a lack of evidence as to the precise value of most elements of the examination, and no evidence as to their predictive value in a general practice population. A questionnaire designed in an American headache centre to screen for temporomandibular disorders found high sensitivity and specificity (92% and 91% respectively) for pain with maximum jaw opening using passive stretch and reciprocal jaw clicking or pain on palpitation over TMJ, to distinguish TMJ derangement from headache patients.[19] One case control study in a headache centre found that papilloedema was an uncommon sign in acute elevation of intracranial pressure.[20]

Investigation

If a headache conforms to the diagnostic criteria of the IHS, there is little value in imaging techniques such as CT scan or MRI. Frishberg[21] reviewed the literature concerning the putative associations between various headache types and intra-cranial pathology, and the literature pertaining to neuroimaging. He concluded that intracranial pathology was rare in patients whose headaches fitted IHS or other accepted criteria. In patients thought to have migraine he recommended imaging as follows: in patients with onset after the age of 60, mental or personality changes, bruits, focal neurology, history of seizures, or those with hemiplegic, basilar or ophthalmoplegic migraine. In cases with onset after the age of 40, no family his-tory, change in pattern, prolonged aura, side-locked headache and resistance to treatment imaging should be considered, but these cases are likely to have very low yield. In the case of headaches other than migraine or cluster headache, he concluded that the literature does not provide enough data to make statistically predictive observations in patients with headache but no findings on neurological examination.

Laboratory investigations such as Hb, CRP and ESR are suggested when the diagnosis of temporal arteritis is suspected. However, evidence from the literature is conflicting. One retrospective study of patients referred for biopsy found no significant difference in either parameter in biopsy-positive or biopsy-negative cases.[22] However, a study using controls as well as the group referred for biopsy found a sensitivity of 100% for CRP, 92% for ESR and the combination of ESR and CRP was highly specific (97%) for temporal arteritis.[11]

Referral (indicator 1)

The Referral Guidelines for Suspected Brain Tumour suggest that a referral should be made and patient seen within 2 weeks for:

▷ subacute progressive focal neurological deficit (e.g. weakness, sensory loss, dysphasia, ataxia)

▷ new-onset seizures characterised by one or more of
 — focal seizures
 — prolonged (greater than 1 hour) post-ictal deficit
 — status epilepicus
 — associated interictal focal deficit

▷ patients with headache, vomiting <u>and</u> papilloedema,

▷ cranial nerve palsy (e.g diplopia, visual failure including optician-defined visual field loss, unilateral sensorineural deafness).

Urgent referral should be considered for

▷ headache patients with non-migrainous headaches of recent onset, present for at least 1 month, when accompanied by features suggestive of raised intracranial pressure (e.g woken by headache, vomiting, drowsiness)

Treatment

This section deals with the evidence for the treatment of primary headache. We have confined our comments to therapeutic agents likely to be used in a UK primary care context. Experts comment on the importance of eliminating triggers, that stress can precipitate any type of headache and that non-drug treatment such as relaxation should be considered.

In the case of migraine, treatment options vary as to the severity of the acute attack. Limmroth et al.[23] reviewed the use of aspirin (acetylsalicylic acid or ASA) in acute treatment and prophylactic treatment of migraine. In the acute phase its effectiveness is enhanced by an effervescent form and combination with antiemetics (of note perhaps is that the dose of ASA used in studies had been of the order of 900 mg). In a multicentre trial, water-soluble aspirin with metoclopramide was as effective as 100 mg of oral sumatriptan in reducing headache intensity and autonomic features such as nausea, and it had fewer adverse effects.[24] Ibuprofen, naproxen and diclofenac sodium have been shown to be effective treatments for an acute attack [25-27] 50 mg of oral diclofenac K provided more rapid relief than oral sumatriptan in a double-blind randomised crossover trial.[28] (The potassium salt is more rapidly absorbed than the sodium.)

Triptan use is recommended for moderate or severe migraine. A systematic review found that subcutaneous sumatriptan was more efficacious than the oral form and had a quicker onset of action, but caused more side-effects.[29] The investigator stated that the majority of side-effects were minor and may be tolerable to patients. A prospective study of the tolerability of subcutaneous sumatriptan in acute migraine, which followed 12 239 patients over 12 months, found no major adverse effects when sumatriptan was used according to the precautions and warnings on the label.[30]

There is evidence from randomised controlled trials for the effectiveness of intramuscular chlorpromazine, metoclopramide and prochlorperazine for an acute attack.[31,32]

Overuse of most acute attack therapies can aggravate headache frequency, and particular care needs to be taken with codeine-containing compound analgesics.

Prophylactic treatment is suggested if attacks occur frequently, or if attacks severely incapacitate the patient (indicator 2). Traditionally, experts have suggested that prophylaxis should be considered if a patient suffers 2 attacks or more each month, but more effective remedies for the acute attack may vary this. The efficacy of commonly used prophylactic drugs is low.[33]

There is clinical trial evidence for the effectiveness of the following drugs in prophylaxis (only propanolol and pitozifen are licensed for migraine prophylaxis in the UK): beta-blockers (atenolol, metoprolol, naldolol, propanolol);[34-36] calcium channel blockers (verapamil, flunarizine);[37,38] serotonin receptor antagonists (pizotifen, methysergide);[39,40] tricyclics (amitriptyline);[41] and 'antiepileptics' (sodium valproate, valproaic acid)[42,43] (indicator 3).

There is evidence for the effectiveness of naproxen but the expert recommendation is to confine its use to the prophylaxis of perimenstrual migraine as intermittent use results in fewer gastrointestinal side-effects.[44,45] Expert opinion is that failure of one beta-blocker does not necessarily predict the response to another. Treatment should start with a low dose and titrate upwards; once pain is controlled, the dose may be tapered down.

In the treatment of headache other than migraine, aspirin and ibuprofen have been shown to be effective in the treatment of episodic tension-type headache.[46] Dosage may be important: a double-blind placebo-controlled comparison of ketoprofen 25 mg and paracetamol 1000 mg found that both were more effective than placebo, with no significant difference between the active agents;[47] and a comparison of ibuprofen 400 mg with paracetamol 1000 mg found ibuprofen to be the more effective.[48] Tricyclics have been found to be effective in reducing the frequency and severity of chronic tension-type headaches.[49]

There is randomised controlled trial evidence for the effect of spinal manipulation in the case of cervicogenic headache.[50] However, spinal manipulation does not have a positive effect on episodic tension-type headache.[51]

Certain prophylactic agents should not be prescribed in specific at-risk groups, for example sumatriptan for patients with angina and beta-blockers for asthmatics (indicator 4).

Follow-up

Experts recommend the use of headache diaries in the assessment and treatment of headache.[9,52] Prophylactic treatment also requires regular monitoring.

Headache in children and adolescents

The diagnosis and treatment of headache in children is broadly similar to that in adults. The criteria for the diagnosis of migraine in children is different, in part relating to aspects of the headache itself, but also noting the difficulty that children may have in articulating characteristics such as the intensity and the nature of pain.[53] Mortimer et al.[54] interviewed children registered at one general practice. Headache prevalence increased from the age of 3 years up to age 11 in boys and girls, with a higher prevalence in 3 to 5-year-old boys than 3 to 5-year-old girls. The overall prevalence of headache was 38.8%, and of migraine was 3.7%. There is a suggestion that tension-type headache in children is associated with psychosocial problems, but the evidence from the literature is conflicting.[55] The history and examination should be supplemented by a developmental assessment. Simple analgesia such as paracetamol is suggested, used early and in adequate dosage (Committee on Safety of Medicines advice is to avoid the use of aspirin in children under 12 years, except for specific indications, due to the risk of Reye's syndrome). Metoclopramide can cause severe extrapyramidal side-effects in children. Zolmitriptan is licensed for use from the age of 12. Pizotifen is used for prophylaxis.

Recommended quality indicators for headache

Diagnosis/referral
1 Patients should be referred urgently for specialist care and investigation if the presenting headache is accompanied by:
   a. suspected raised intracranial pressure
   b. new-onset seizure
   c. focal neurological signs
   d. papilloedema

Treatment
2 Prophylaxis treatment should be offered in patients with severe and disabling migraine
3 The following agents should be prescribed as first line for prophylaxis of migraine unless contraindicated:
   a. beta-blocker
   b. tricyclic antidepressant
   c. pizotifen
4 a. Sumatriptan should not be prescribed for migraine in patients with angina
   b. Beta-blockers should not be prescribed for migraine in patients with asthma

---

Overview of data sources used in this review

Articles on headache were identified by a search of the 1991–5 and 1996–9 Medline databases and the Cochrane library. Keywords in the search were 'headache' (exploded and used as textword), 'family practice', 'epidemiology', 'sensitivity and specificity', and 'treatment'. We searched particularly for literature with a community/general practice focus. However, the majority of evidence is from specialist centres and uses the classification of headache of The International Headache Society (IHS).[56] This establishes diagnostic criteria for headache using a hierarchical scale and has been used since 1988 for epidemiological and clinical research.[56] Guidelines for the diagnosis and management of headache and migraine have been produced by a number of groups and these were also reviewed.[57, 58] Migraine management guidelines have been produced by the British Association for the Study of Headache[59] and a group endorsed by Migraine in Primary Care Advisors.[60] Referral Guidelines for Suspected Brain Tumours have been prepared as part of the initiative to allow patients with suspected cancer to be seen by a specialist within 2 weeks.

There is an absence of evidence relating to the management of headache in primary care practice and many aspects of diagnosis and treatment are based on expert opinion.

Further reading

Goadsby Peter J, Olesen Jes. Fortnightly review: diagnosis and management of migraine. *British Medical Journal* 1996; 312: 1279–1283

Pryse-Phillips WE, Dodick DW, Edmeads JC et al. Guidelines for the diagnosis and management of migraine in clinical practice. *Canadian Medical Association Journal* 1997; 156: 1273–1287

The British Association for the Study of Headache (BASH) has a website at www.bash.org.uk

References

1. Rasmussen BK, Jensen R, Schroll M, Olesen J. Epidemiology of headache in a general population – a prevalence study. Journal of Clinical Epidemiology 1991; 44(11): 1147–1157
2. Lipton RB, Stewart WF. The epidemiology of migraine. European Neurology 1994; 34(suppl 2): 6–11
3. Rasmussen BK. Epidemiology of headache. Cephalalgia 1995; 15: 45–68
4. Jensen R. Pathophysiological mechanisms of tension type headache: a review of epidemiological and experimental studies. Cephalalgia 1999; 19: 602–621
5. Scher AI, Stewart WF, Liberman J, Lipton RB. Prevalence of frequent headache in a population sample. Headache 1998; 38: 497–506
6. Castillo J, Munoz P, Guitera V, Pascual J. Epidemiology of chronic daily headache in the general population. Headache 1999; 39: 190–196
7. Royal College of General Practitioners, Office of Populations Censuses and Surveys, Department of Health. Morbidity statistics in general practice fourth national study 1991–1992. London: HMSO, 1995
8. Cockerell OC, Goodridge DMG, Brodie D, Sander JWAS, Shorvon SD. Neurological disease in a defined population: the results of a pilot study in two general practices. Neuroepidemiology 1996; 15: 73–82
9. Goadsby Peter J, Olesen J. Fortnightly review: diagnosis and management of migraine. British Medical Journal 1996; 312: 1279–1283
10. Gervil M, Ulrich V, Olesen J, Russell MB. Screening for migraine in the general population: validation of a simple questionnaire. Cephalalgia 1998; 18: 342–348
11. Hayreh SS, Podhajsky PA, Raman R, Zimmerman B. Giant cell arteritis: validity and reliabiity of various diagnostic tests. American Journal of Ophthalmology 1997; 123(3): 285–296
12. Attia J, Hatala R, Cook DJ, Wong JG. Does this adult patient have acute meningitis? Journal of the American Medical Association 1999; 282: 175–181
13. Breslau N, Schultz LR, Stewart WF, Lipton RB, Lucia VC, Welch KMA. Headache and major depression. Is the association specific to migraine? Neurology 2000; 54: 308–313
14. Holroyd K A, Stensland M, Lipchik, GL, Hill, KR, O'Donnell FS, Cordingley G. Psychosocial correlates and impact of chronic tension-type headaches. Headache 2000; 40: 3–16
15. Mitsikostas DD, Thomas AM. Comorbidity of headache and depressive disorders. Cephalalgia 1999; 19: 211–217
16. Wang SJ, Liu HC, Fuh JL, Liu CY, Wang PN, Lu SR. Comorbidity of headache and depression in the elderly. Pain 1999; 82(3): 239–243
17. Ham LP, Andrasik F, Packard RC, Bundrick CM. Psychopathology in individuals with post-traumatic headache and other pain types. Cephalalgia 1994; 14: 118–126
18. Marks DR, Papoport AM. Practical evaluation and diagnosis of headache. Seminars in Neurology 1997; 17(4): 307–312
19. Schiffman E, Haley D, Baker C, Lindgren B. Diagnostic criteria for screening headache patients for temporomandibular disorders. Headache 1995; 35: 121–124
20. Steffen H, Eifert B, Aschoff A, Kolling GH, Volcker HE. The diagnostic value of optic disc evaluation in acute elevated intracranial pressure. Ophthalmology 1996; 103(8): 1229–1232
21. Frishberg B. Neuroimaging in presumed primary headache disorders. Seminars in Neurology 1997; 17 (4): 373–382
22. Chmelewski WL, McKnight KM, Agudelo CA, Wise CM. Presenting features and outcomes in patients undergoing temporal artery biopsy. Archives of Internal Medicine 1992; 152: 1690–1695
23. Limmroth V, Katsarva Z, Diener H-C. Acetylsalicylic acid in the treatment of headache. Cephalalgia 1999; 19: 545–551
24. Tfelt-Hansen P, Henry P, Mulder LJ, Schneidewaert RG, Schoenen J, Chazot G. The effectiveness of combined oral lysine acetylsalicylate and metoclopramide compared with oral sumatriptan for migraine. Lancet 1995; 346: 923–926
25. Treves TA, Streiffler M, Korezyn AD. Naproxen sodium versus ergotamine tartrate in the treatment of acute migraine attacks. Headache 1992; 32(6): 280–282

26. Karachalios Gn, Fotiadou A, Nickolaos C, Karabetsos A, Kehagioglou K. Treatment of acute migraine attack with diclofenac sodium: a double-blind study. Headache 1992; 32: 98–100
27. Kloster R, Nestvold K, Vilming ST. A double-blind study of ibuprofen versus placebo in the treatment of acute migraine attacks. Cephalalgia 1992; 12: 169–171
28. Diclofenac-K/Sumatriptan Migraine Study Group. Acute treatment of migraine: efficacy and safety of a non-steroidal anti-inflammatory drug, diclofenac-potassium in comparison to oral sumatriptan and placebo Cephalalgia 1999; 19: 232–240
29. Tfelt-Hansen P. Efficay and adverse effects of subcutaneous, oral and intranasal sumatriptan used for migraine treatment: a systematic review based on number needed to treat. Cephalalgia 1998; 18: 532–538
30. O'Quinn S, Davis RL, Gutterman DL, Pait GD, Fox AW. Prospective large-scale study of the tolerability of subcutaneous sumatriptan injection for the acute treatment of migraine. Cephalalgia 1999; 19: 223–231
31. Lane PL, McLellan BA, Baggoley CJ. Comparative efficacy of chlorpromazine and meperidine with dimenhydrinate in migraine headache. Annals of Emergency Medicine 1989; 18(4): 360–365
32. Coppola M, Yealy DM, Laibold RA. Randomised, placebo controlled evaluation of prochlorperazine versus metoclopramide for emergency department treatment of migraine headaches. Annals of Emergency Medicine 1995; 26: 541–546
33. Ramadan NM, Schultz LL, Gilkey SJ. Migraine prophylactic drugs: proof of efficacy, utilization and cost. Cephalalgia 1997; 17(2): 73–80
34. Johannsson V, Nilsson LR, Widelius T et al. Atenolol in migraine prophylaxis: a double blind cross over multicentre study. Headache 1987; 27: 372–4
35. Gerber WD, Diener H C, Scholz E, Nierderberger U. Responders and non-responders to metoprolol, propanolol and nifedipine treatment in migraine prophylaxis: a dose range study based on time series analysis. Cephalalgia 1991; 11: 37–45
36. Ryan Sr RE, Ryan Jr RE, Sudilovsky A. Nadolol: its use in the prophylactic treatment of migraine. Headache 1983; 23: 26–31
37. Markley HG. Verapamil and migraine prophylaxis: mechanisms and efficacy. American Journal of Medicine 1991; 90(suppl 5A): 48S–53S
38. Soelberg Sorensen P, Larsen BH, Rasmussen MJK, Kinge E, Iversen H. Flunarizine versus metoprolol in migraine prophylaxis: a double blind, randomised parallel group study of efficacy and tolerability. Headache 1991; 31: 650–657
39. Drummond PD. Effectiveness of methysergide in relation to clinical features of migraine. Headache 1985; 5: 145–146
40. Capildeo R, Rose FC. Single dose pizotifen, 1.5 mg nocte: a new approach in the prophylaxis of migraine. Headache 1982; 22: 272–275
41. Bank J. A comparative study of amitriptyline and fluvoxamine in migraine prophylaxis. Headache 1994; 34: 476–478
42. Herring R, Kuritzky RS. Sodium valproate in the prophylactic treatment of migraine: a double blind study versus placebo. Cephalalgia 1992; 12: 81–84
43. Jensen R, Brinck T, Olesen J. Prophylactic effect of sodium valproate in migraine without aura: a double-blind, placebo- and dose-controlled study. Cephalalgia 1993; 13(13): 193
44. Welch KMA, Ellis DJ, Keenan PA. Successful migraine prophylaxis with naproxen sodium. Neurology 1985; 35: 1304–1310
45. Szekely B, Merryman S, Croft H, Post G. Prophylactic effects of naproxen sodium on perimenstrual headache: a double blind placebo controlled study. Cephalalgia 1989; 9 (suppl 10): 452–453
46. Nebe J, Heier M, Diener HC. Low dose ibuprofen in self medication of mild to moderate headache: a comparison with acetylsaliscylic acid and placebo. Cephalalgia 1995; 15: 531–535
47. Steiner TJ, Lange R. Ketoprofen (25 mg) in the symptomatic treatment of episodic tension type headache: double-blind placebo-controlled comparison with acetaminophen (1000 g). Cephalalgia 1998; 18(1): 38–43
48. Schachtel BP, Furey SA, Thoden WR. Non-prescription ibuprofen and acetaminophen in the treatment of tension-type headache. Journal of Clinical Pharmacology 1996; 36 (12): 1120–1125
49. Bendtsen L, Jensen R, Olesen J. A non-selective (amitriptyline), but not a selective (citalopram), serotonin reuptake inhibitor is effective in the prophylactic treatment of chronic tension-type headache. Journal of Neurology, Neurosurgery and Psychiatry 1996; 61(3): 285–290
50. Nilsson NA, Christenson HW, Hartvigsan J. The effect of spinal manipulation in the treatment of cervicogenic headache. Journal of Manipulative and Physiological Therapeutics 1997; 20: 326–330
51. Bove G, Nilsson N (1998) Spinal manipulation in the treatment of episodic tension-type headache: a randomised controlled trial. Journal of the American Medical Association 1998; 280: 1576–1579

52. Russell MB, Rasmussen BK, Brennum J, Iversen HK, Jensen RA, Olesen J. Presentation of a new instrument: the diagnostic headache diary. Cephalalgia 1992; 12: 369–374

53. Lipton RB. Diagnosis and epidemiology of pediatric migraine. Current Opinion in Neurology 1997; 10: 231–236

54. Mortimer J, Kay J, Jaron A. Epidemiology of headache and childhood migraine in an urban general practice using ad hoc, Vahiquist and IHS criteria. Developmental Medicine and Child Neurology 1992; 34: 1095–1101

55. Karwautz A, Wober C, Lang T et al. Psychosocial factors in children and adolescents with migraine and tension type headache: a controlled study and review of the literature. Cephalalgia 1999; 19: 32–43

56. Headache Classification Committee of the International Headache Society. Classification and diagnostic criteria for headache disorders, cranial neuralgias and facial pain. Cephalalgia 1988; 8 (suppl 7)

57. Pryse-Phillips WE, Dodick DW, Edmeads JC et al. Guidelines for the diagnosis and management of migraine in clinical practice. Canadian Medical Association Journal 1997; 156: 1273–1287

58. Danish Neurological Society and Danish Headache Society. Guidelines for the management of headache. Cephalalgia 1998; 18: 9–22

59. British Association for the Study of Headache. Guidelines for all doctors in the diagnosis and management of migraine. London: Princess Margaret Migraine Clinic, 1999

60. Migraine in Primary Care Advisors. Migraine management guidelines. Synergy Medical Education, 1997

16

Upper respiratory tract infections

Paul Little

Importance

Acute upper respiratory tract infections (URTIs) are the commonest reason for patients to seek medical advice[1] and also the commonest reason for antibiotics to be prescribed. The current major concern is that the inappropriate use of antibiotics for usually self-limiting conditions will foster the development of antibiotic resistance and lead to serious infections becoming untreatable.[2-6] For this reason it is currently a national priority not to encourage the use of antibiotics unless there is very good evidence of their efficacy.

Pharyngitis/tonsillitis: diagnosis

Pharyngitis is caused by both bacterial and viral organisms.[7] Antibiotics could be targeted to those who have positive throat swabs for group A Streptococcus, a positive rapid Strep. test, or clinical characteristics associated with a positive throat swab.[8-11] Alternatively throat swabs could be used in selected populations.[11] However, throat swabs increase costs significantly, potentially medicalise self-limiting illness[12] and rarely modify clinical decisions.[13] In addition, antibiotic use and overall accuracy of decision making may be unchanged.[14] The throat swab is neither particularly sensitive nor specific when compared to a rise in antistreptolysin-O titres (ASOT). This is the case in both the general population[15] and in selected general practice populations where clinical selection has occurred.[16] Clinical scores or decision rules based on the throat swab[8-11] have the same limitations of validity as the throat swab, although they may crudely identify patients at risk of complications (see below).

Pharyngitis/tonsillitis: treatment

Antibiotics

A systematic review[17] indicates that antibiotics reduce symptom duration by a few hours to half a day. For patients who are not systemically unwell, either not prescribing or using a delayed prescribing approach (waiting for several days before using the prescription) is acceptable, changes attitudes to antibiotics, modifies attendance behaviour and does not delay symptom resolution appreciably.[18,19] Delaying the prescription probably results in 20% fewer recurrences compared to the immediate prescriptions of antibiotics, presumably because antibiotics modify local or systemic immune mechanisms.[20-22]

For the commoner complications, such as otitis media, 30 children and 140 adults would have to be treated to prevent 1 case of otitis media, which is a self-limiting illness anyway.[17] For the rarer complications (rheumatic fever) the evidence of efficacy is based on highly atypical populations.[17] The commonest major suppurative complication is quinsy, which has an incidence of about 1 in 400 following presentation to the doctor with sore throat in patients who are not systemically unwell[18,19] and a similar incidence from routine data.[23,24] The systematic review[17] relies for most of its data (providing 76% of the weighting) on an old study of patients admitted to hospital, when the prevalence of quinsy in untreated patients was very high (1:18). Quinsy following sore throat is more common (1:60) in unwell patients with 3 out of 4 Centor criteria,[9] most of whom have fever.[25] In such patients two 'efficacy' trials suggest that quinsy may be prevented with oral penicillin.[25,26] However, the effectiveness of penicillin in preventing quinsy in practice is not likely to be 100% as these two trials would suggest, since in the routine setting compliance is not rigorously assessed as it is in efficacy trials: routine data suggest that many patients develop quinsy despite the use of penicillin.[24]

Whether using the clinical Centor criteria is better than GPs' assessment of how unwell patients are is unclear. Where a GP feels that a patient is not very unwell systemically the rate of quinsy is low, and the patient can be safely offered no prescription or a delayed prescription.[18,19] Thus for clinical presentations where the GP judges a patient to be both systemically unwell (i.e. not the low-risk group) and to have 3 out of 4 of the Centor criteria (i.e. the higher risk group), it would be reasonable to treat with penicillin or at least discuss with the patient the likely risks of non-treatment – but patients may still feel that a 1:60 chance of developing quinsy does not make it worth taking a course of antibiotics.

If an antibiotic is prescribed, then a narrow-spectrum antibiotic (penicillin V) will minimise both side-effects and the risk of resistance. A 10-day course will better eradicate *Streptococcus*,[27-30] but the clinical significance of this is unclear. Longer courses also have the disadvantage of poorer compliance, and possibly greater likelihood of antibiotic resistance. Twice-daily dosing results in better compliance, and better clinical and microbiological outcomes.[31] Amoxycillin or ampicillin will cause a rash in patients with glandular fever, so erythromycin can be used where penicillin allergy has been documented (indicator 2)

Treatment of patients with rheumatic fever
Trial evidence from atypical settings supports treating patients with a past history of rheumatic fever in order to prevent further attacks[17] (indicator 1).

Other medical treatments
Treatment with aspirin in children is contraindicated due to the avoidable risk of Reye's syndrome. The incidence of Reye's syndrome has dramatically reduced since the discovery of its association with aspirin and the subsequent reduction in aspirin use, as publicised[32] (indicator 3). Non steroidal anti-inflammatory drugs (NSAIDs) are helpful[33-40] but have not been shown to be better than paracetamol.[33] Benzydamine hydrochloride gargle may also help symptoms.[41]

Lower respiratory tract infection: diagnosis

Acute lower respiratory tract infection (LRTI) can be defined as a cough of less than 3 weeks duration with another symptom (sputum, short of breath, pain) or generalised signs localising to the lower tract, and without other lung pathology.[42-44] Most bronchitis is due to viruses, but several bacteria have been implicated.

The absence of vital sign abnormality or localised abnormality on examination of the chest make pneumonia very unlikely.[45] In children the best sign for predicting pneumonia is tachypnoea, and if all clinical signs (respiratory rate, auscultation, work of breathing) are normal (indicator 4), CXR findings are unlikely to be positive.[46] Routine x-ray is not likely to affect outcome[47] and since it will not alter management decisions or outcome in most cases, it cannot be routinely recommended in acute illness.

Lower respiratory tract infection: treatment

Antibiotics

The mixed evidence from published systematic reviews and the small size of the reviews[48-50] suggests that more evidence is needed. Furthermore, patients who were very systemically unwell are unlikely to have been included in these studies, and the reviews were not large enough to assess whether treatment prevents complications. However, until more evidence is available, the equivocal existing evidence combined with the national priority to minimise prescribing antibiotics supports a strategy of no immediate prescription of antibiotics for uncomplicated LRTI (indicator 5).

Bronchodilators and corticosteroids

A systematic review did not support the use of anticholinergic therapy for young children who wheeze with respiratory tract infections.[51] For school-age children without asthma who had an URTI and wheeze, inhaled corticosteroid produced a modest improvement in FEV1 but did not shorten the illness.[52] Oral ß-agonists have shown mixed results in patients with acute cough, and they have significant side-effects,[53,54] but a metered dose inhaler may help.[55,56] Nebulised sodium cromoglycate has demonstrated mixed results in children with 'wheezy bronchitis'.[57,58]

Other treatments

Antitussives,[59-61] mucolytics[62-64] and NSAIDs[65] may help symptomatically. Providing an information leaflet reduces reattendance,[66] probably by modifying patient expectations about the natural history of LRTI.

Nasal congestion and rhinorrhoea: treatment

Symptomatic

Oral decongestants,[67,68] topical decongestants[69] and intranasal ipratropium bromide[70] are probably effective whereas saline or medicated nosedrops are probably not effective.[71,72] Evidence of rhinitis medicamentosa starts to develop at 10 days with topical decongestants:[73] thus the BNF (British National Formulary) guidelines of a maximum of 7 days seem reasonable. Care should be taken with oral decongestants in patients with heart disease and hypertension, due to the moderate systemic effects.[74] A systematic review suggests that steam may also provide some relief of symptoms.[75]

Antibiotics

A systematic review suggests that antibiotics for the common cold are not likely to be helpful.[76] The expert panels did not want to be proscriptive and therefore suggested an indicator allowing antibiotics to be prescribed if the symptoms persisted for longer than 14 days (indicator 6).

Other treatments

A review of trials identified from a search of reviews indicates little benefit of antihistamines for colds.[77] A systematic review of zinc lozenges[78] suggests that they may produce marginal benefit at 1 week, but there is concern about the considerable heterogeneity of the available trials. A systematic review of the herbal product echinacea[79] demonstrated positive results in most studies, but there was not enough evidence to recommend the use of a specific echinacea product. Intranasal sodium cromoglycate[80,81] and NSAIDs[82] may also help.

Influenza: diagnosis

There are approximately 0.50 episodes per person year of influenza in western countries.[83] Most cases are caused by the influenza A virus which is dispersed by sneezing, coughing or talking. Although influenza causes several complications and pandemics cause a heavy death toll,[28,84] most adults under the age of 50 are at low risk of complications.

Uncomplicated influenza has an abrupt onset of systemic symptoms including fever, chills, headache and myalgia. The fever lasts for 3–4 days normally but can persist for up to 7 days. Respiratory symptoms (e.g. cough, hoarseness, nasal discharge, pharyngitis) begin when systemic symptoms begin to resolve. The best clinical predictors of serologically confirmed influenza in 1838 patients were acute onset, fever and cough.[85] Dyspnoea, haemoptysis, wheezing, purulent sputum, fever persisting more than 7 days, severe muscle pain and dark urine may indicate the onset of influenza complications.[28]

Influenza: treatment

Treatment for uncomplicated influenza is generally symptomatic, with rest, fluid intake and aspirin or paracetamol. There is evidence that NSAIDs are no more effective than aspirin for symptoms of influenza.[86,87]

Amantadine and rimantadine decrease virus shedding and shorten the duration of fever by approximately 1 day if started within 48 hours of the onset of symptoms.[88] Amantadine and rimantadine also prevent influenza.[88] However, both cause significant side-effects and it is unclear how much extra benefit is provided when patients are taking full doses of paracetamol and aspirin/NSAIDs. It is also unclear whether the use of these agents can be justified economically. Furthermore, the generalisability of the evidence for treatment and prevention is unclear: most subjects included in the trials were volunteers, medical students or military personnel.

Influenza: prevention

Observational studies demonstrate that vaccination probably reduces the risk of respiratory illness, pneumonia, hospitalisation and death in those over the age of 65[89] and for the chronically ill.[90] A small systematic review of vaccination for patients with asthma[91] concluded that there was not enough evidence to assess the benefits and risks of influenza vaccination. This review was conducted and the indicators rated before the recent guidelines on immunisation against influenza were produced by the National Institute for Clinical Excellence.

Acute sinusitis: diagnosis

Acute sinusitis is normally defined as an infection with a duration of less than 3 weeks and is an uncommon complication of URTI.[17] Many patients with facial pain and tenderness will not have sinusitis and it is difficult to determine what clinical symptoms and signs best predict sinusitis. Sinus puncture is perhaps the best 'gold' standard since it indicates the presence of infecting organisms, although contamination by commensal organism can occur. Other standards such as CT and MRI will show evidence of thickened mucosa and fluid, but cannot indicate whether this is due to infection or inflammation and there have been no studies comparing CT with sinus puncture. A sinus radiograph is reasonably sensitive (73%) and specific (80%) compared with sinus puncture.[92] Using 4-view x-ray as the standard, a history of purulent nasal discharge, maxillary toothache, purulent secretions on examination, poor response to decongestants and abnormal illumination of the sinuses are predictive of sinusitis: 4 or more symptoms or signs have a likelihood ratio of a positive test of 6.[93,94] However, sinus illumination is likely to be operator or setting dependent.[95]

The presence of fluid and total opacification of the sinuses on CT predict antibiotic response.[96] A study using CT as the gold standard documented similar findings to the x-ray studies: purulent rhinorrhoea, purulent secretion in the cavum nasae, a history of double sickening (getting better, then getting worse again) and an ESR of greater than 10 are predictive of a CT diagnosis of sinusitis. Three out of the 4 had a likelihood ratio of a positive test of 1.8.[97] However, a 4-item clinical risk score – purulent rhinorrhoea with unilateral predominance, local pain with unilateral predominance, bilateral purulent rhinorrhoea, and presence of pus in the nasal cavity – is likely to be as sensitive and specific as any other method in predicting results of sinus puncture.[98]

Acute sinusitis: treatment

Antibiotics

Traditionally 10–14 days of antibiotics have been advocated, but a systematic review suggests that the absolute benefit for symptom resolution is moderate.[99] Furthermore, most studies in general practice show moderate or no effect.[100–104]

Decongestants and antihistamines

Topical decongestants probably do not help x-ray changes or symptoms.[105,106] If topical decongestants are used, the *BNF* guidelines of a maximum of 7 days are reasonable. Antihistamines may be helpful for patients with sinusitis who have a history of allergic rhinitis.[107]

Other treatments

There is mixed evidence for the use of topical steroids.[108-110] NSAIDs are likely to be helpful,[111,112] but they may not be significantly more effective than paracetamol.[111] Proteolytics and mucolytics may also help.[113-116]

Chronic sinusitis: diagnosis

Sinusitis that has continued for more than 3 months is classified as chronic. It generally presents with dull facial ache or pressure (sometimes worse in the morning and with head movement) with nasal congestion, thick pharyngeal secretions, blocked ears, dental pain, chronic cough, mild facial swelling and eye pain.[117] Diagnosis as with acute sinusitis is initially by history and examination (see acute sinusitis): investigations that can be considered to confirm the diagnosis (but with the limitations outlined in acute sinusitis) are 4-view x-ray, nasal endoscopy (the most specific) or CT scanning (less specific, but can demonstrate underlying sinus disease). Lasar et al.[118] evaluated radiographs and CT scans compared to intraoperative findings and showed that CT performed much better in chronic sinusitis regarding diagnosis and evaluation of the need for surgery. However, investigation other than x-ray would not normally be arranged in primary care, and treatment and referral are more likely to be based on history and examination and/or x-ray.

Chronic sinusitis: treatment

Antibiotics

Antibiotics may not work better than sinus lavage for children,[119] and neither antibiotics nor drainage are curative in children.[120] In a small study of both adults and

---

Recommended quality indicators for upper respiratory tract infections

Tonsillopharyngitis
1 Patients with a documented past history of rheumatic fever presenting with tonsillitis or pharyngitis should be advised to take a course of antibiotics unless contraindicated or intolerant
2 If throat infections are treated, treatment should be with penicillin V unless the patient is allergic to penicillin
3 Aspirin should not be prescribed or advised for children with URTIs under the age of 12 years

Bronchitis
4 Patients with the following symptoms should receive a physical examination of their chest:
   a. acute cough with fever persisting for 1 week or deteriorating
   b. acute cough with shortness of breath
5 An antibiotic prescription should not be offered to patients with uncomplicated bronchitis with symptoms of fewer than 14 days duration

Rhinitis
6 An antibiotic prescription should not be offered to patients with uncomplicated infective rhinitis with symptoms of fewer than 14 days duration

---

children, clarithromycin performed better than erythromycin,[121] and ciprofloxacin does not perform significantly better than amoxycillin/clavulanic acid.[122]

Other treatments

Topical steroids,[123] decongestants[124] and immune stimulants may also help.[125,126]

Overview of data sources used in this review

This review is based on a search of the Cochrane library database of systematic reviews and trials using the disease terms 'influenza', 'pharyngitis', 'tonsillitis', 'bronchitis', 'rhinitis' and 'sinusitis' and a search of Medline 1989–9 using the same terms (exploded) and diagnosis (subheadings: adverse effects, classification, statistics and numerical data, education, standards, history, instrumentation, utilization, methods).

References

1. HMSO, OPCS. Morbidity statistics from general practice: fourth national study 1991. London: HMSO, 1994
2. Arason V, Kristinsson K, Sigurdsson J, Stefansdottir G, Molstad S, Gudmundsson S. Do antimicrobials increase the rate of penicillin resistant pneumococci in children? Cross sectional prevalence study. British Medical Journal 1996; 313: 387–391
3. Magee J, Pritchard E. Antibiotic prescribing and antibiotic resistance in community practice: retrospective study. British Medical Journal 1999; 319: 1239–1240
4. Seppala H, Klaukka T, Vuopio-Varkila J. The effect of changes in the consumption of macrolide antibiotics on erythromycin resistance in group A Streptococci. New England Journal of Medicine 1997; 337: 441–446
5. House of Lords. House of Lords Select Committee on Science and Technology: 7th report. Occasional Report 1998
6. SMAC. Standing Medical Advisory Committee (SMAC) report: the path of least resistance. Occasional Report 1998
7. Hammerschlag M. Pharyngitis. In: Oski F, ed. Principles and practice of pediatrics. Philadelphia: Lippincott, 1994: 969–970
8. Dobbs F. A scoring system for predicting group A streptococcal throat infection. British Journal of General Practice 1996; 46: 461–464
9. Centor RM, Witherspoon JM, Dalton HP. The diagnosis of strep throat in the emergency room. Medical Decision Making 1981; 1: 239–246
10. Breese B. A simple scorecard for the tentative diagnosis of streptococcal pharyngitis. American Journal of Diseases of Children. 1977; 131: 514–517
11. Komaroff A, Pass T, Aronson M, et al. The prediction of streptococcal pharyngitis in adults. Journal of General Internal Medicine 1986; 1: 1–7
12. Kolmos H, Little P. Should general practitioners perform diagnostic tests on patients before prescribing antibiotics? British Medical Journal 1999; 318: 799–802
13. Burke P, Bain J, Lowes A, Athersuch R. Rational decisions and managing sore throat. British Medical Journal 1988; 296: 1646–1649
14. Hedges J, Singal B, Estep J. The impact of a rapid screen for streptococcal pharyngitis on clinical decision making in the emergency department. Medical Decision Making 1991; 11: 119–124
15. Del Mar C. Managing sore throat: a literature review I: making the diagnosis. Medical Journal of Australia 1992; 156: 572–575
16. Dagnelie C, Bartelink M, Van Der Graaf Y, Goessens W, De Melker R. Towards better diagnosis of throat infections with GABHS in general practice. British Journal of General Practice 1998; 48: 959–962
17. Del Mar C, Glaziou P. Antibiotics for the symptoms and complications of sore throat. In: the Cochrane Database of Systematic Reviews. The Cochrane Library, last amended May 1998:

18. Little PS, Williamson I, Warner G, Gould C, Gantley M, Kinmonth AL. An open randomised trial of prescribing strategies for sore throat. British Medical Journal 1997; 314: 722–727

19. Little PS, Gould C, Williamson.I., Warner G, Gantley M, Kinmonth AL. Reattendance and complications in a randomised trial of prescribing strategies for sore throat: the medicalising effect of prescribing antibiotics. British Medical Journal 1997; 315: 350–352

20. Pichichero ME, Disney F, Talpey W et al. Adverse and beneficial effects of immediate treatment of group A beta haemolytic streptococcal pharyngitis. Pediatric Infectious Disease Journal 1987; 6: 635–643

21. Gerber M, Randolph M, DeMeo K, Kaplan E. Lack of impact of early antibiotic therapy for streptococcal pharyngitis on recurrence rates. Journal of Pediatrics 1990; 117: 853–858

22. El-Daher N, Hijazi S, Rawashdeh N, Al-Kalil I, Abu-Ektaish F, Abdel-Latif D. Immediate versus delayed treatment of Group A beta-haemolytic streptococcal pharyngitis with penicillin V. Pediatric Infectious Disease Journal 1991; 10: 126–130

23. Little PS, Williamson IW. Sore throat management in general practice. Family Practice 1996; 13(3): 317–321

24. Simo R, Avinash P, Belloso A et al. Complications of sore throat are not rare. British Medical Journal 1998; 316: 631

25. Zwart S, Sachs A, Ruijs G, Hoes A, DeMelker R. Penicillin for acute sore throat: randomised double blind trial of seven days versus three days treatment or placebo in adults. British Medical Journal 2000; 320: 150–154

26. Dagnelie CF, Van der Graf Y, De Melker R, Touw-Otten FWMM. Do patients with sore throat benefit from penicillin? A Randomised double blind placebo controlled clinical trial with penicillin V in general practice. British Journal of General Practice 1996; 46: 589–593

27. Perlman P, Ginn D. Respiratory infections in adults: choosing the best treatment. Postgraduate Medicine 1990; 87: 175–184

28. Barker L, Burton J, Zieve P. Principles of Ambulatory Medicine. Baltimore, MD: Williams & Wilkins, 1991

29. Catanzaro F, Rammelkamp C, Chamovitz R. Prevention of rheumatic fever by treatment of streptococcal infections. New England Journal of Medicine 1958; 259: 51–57

30. Schwartz R, Wientzen R, Pedreira F. Penicillin V for group A streptococcal pharyngotonsillitis: a randomised trial of seven vs ten days therapy. Journal of the American Medical Association 1981; 246: 1790–1795

31. Raz R, Elchanan G, Colodner R et al. Penicillin V twice daily vs four times daily in the treatment of streptococcal pharyngitis. Infectious Diseases in Clinical Practice 1995; 4: 50–54

32. Belay E, Bresee J, Holman R, Khan A, Shariari A, Schonberger L. Reye's syndrome in the United States from 1981 through 1997. New England Journal of Medicine 1999; 340: 1377–1382

33. Bertin L, Pons G, d'Athis P, Maudelonde C, Duhamel J, Olive G. Randomised double blind multicenter controlled trial of ibuprofen versus acetaminophen (paracetamol) and placebo for treatment of the symptoms of tonsillitis and pharyngitis in children. Journal of Pediatrics 1991; 119: 811–814

34. Benarrhosh C. Double-blind multicentric comparative study of tiaprofenic acid in the treatment of children with tonsillitis and pharyngitis. Archives Francaises de Pediatrie 1989; 46: 541–546

35. Sauvage J, Ditisheim A, Bessede J, David N. Double blind placebo controlled multi centre trial of the efficacy and tolerance of niflumic acid capsules in the treatment of tonsillitis in adults. Current Medical Research and Opinion 1990; 11(10): 631–637

36. Nouri M. Nimesulide for treatment of acute inflammation of the upper respiratory tract. Clinical Therapeutics 1984; 6(2): 142–150

37. Manach Y, Ditisheim A. Double blind placebo controlled trial of the efficacy and tolerance of morniflumate suppositories in the treatment of tonsillitis in children. Journal of Internal Medical Research 1990; 18: 30–36

38. Benarrhosh C, Ullmann A. Efficacy and tolerability of tiaprofenic acid in pharyngitis in adults. Presse Medicale 1989; 18: 716–718

39. Vauzelle-Kervroedan F, Revzani Y, Pons G et al. Antipyretic efficacy of tiaprofenic acid in febrile children. Fundamental and Clinical Pharmacology 1996; 10: 56–59

40. Chelly M, Dahan R, Laboyd M, Dupont F, Lacoste C, Larue F. Open controlled trial of the efficacy and tolerability of morniflumate child suppository vs alpha amylase syrup in sore throat. Annales De Pediatrie 1996; 43: 392–402

41. Wethington J. Double blind study of benzydamine hydrochloride, a new treatment for sore throat. Clinical Therapeutics 1985; 7: 641–646

42. Billas A. Lower respiratory tract infections. Primary Care 1990; 17: 811–824

43. Macfarlane JT, Colville A, Guion A. Prospective study of aetiology and outcome of adult lower respiratory tract infections in the community. Lancet 1993; 341: 511–514

44. Pratter M, Bartter T, Akers S, DuBois J. An algorithmic approach to chronic cough. Annals of Internal Medicine 1993; 119: 977–983
45. Metlay J, Kapoor W, Fine M. Does this patient have community acquired pneumonia. Journal of the American Medical Association 1997; 278: 1440–1445
46. Margolis PG. Does this infant have pneumonia? Journal of the American Medical Association 1998; 279: 308–313
47. Swingler G, Zwarenstein M. Chest radiograph in acute respiratory infections in children. Cochrane Library, updated May 1999
48. Fahey T, Stocks N, Thomas T. Quantitative systematic review of randomised controlled trials comparing antibiotics with placebo for acute cough in adults. British Medical Journal 1998; 316: 906–910
49. Fahey T, Stocks N, Thomas T. A systematic review of the treatment of upper respiratory infection in children. Archives of Disease in Childhood 1997; 79(3): 225–230
50. Becker L, Glazier R, McIsaac W, Smucny J. Antibiotics for acute bronchitis. Cochrane Library, updated August 1997
51. Everard M, Kurian M. Anticholinergic drugs for wheeze in children under the age of two years. Cochrane Library 1998
52. Doull I, Lampe F, Smith S, Schreiber J, Freezer N, Holgate S. Effect of inhaled corticosteroid on episodes of wheezing associated with viral infection in school age children: randomised double blind placebo controlled trial. British Medical Journal 1997; 315: 858–862
53. Littenberg B, Wheeler M, Smith D. A randomised controlled trial of oral albuterol in acute cough. Journal of Family Practice 1996; 42: 49–53
54. Hueston W. A comparison of albuterol and erythromycin for the treatment of acute bronchitis. Journal of Family Practice 1991; 33: 476–480
55. Hueston W. Albuterol delivered by metered dose inhaler to treat acute bronchitis. Journal of Family Practice 1994; 39: 437–440
56. Lafortuna C, Fazio F. Acute effect of inhaled salbutamol on mucociliary clearance in health and acute bronchitis. Respiration 1984; 45: 111–123
57. Geller-Bernstein C, Levin S. Nebulised sodium cromoglycate in the treatment of wheezy bronchitis in infants and young children. Respiration 1982; 43: 294–298
58. Bertelsen A, Andersen J, Busch P et al. Nebulised sodium cromoglycate in the treatment of wheezy bronchitis. A multicentre double blind placebo controlled study. Allergy 1986; 41: 266–270
59. Berthelot J, Weibel M. Comparative clinical evaluation of the antitussive activity of butamirate citrate linctus vs a codeine linctus. Clinical Trials Journal 1990; 27: 50–57
60. Gastpar H, Criscuolo D, Dieterich H. Efficacy and tolerability of glaucine as an antitussive agent. Current Medical Research and Opinion 1984; 9: 21–27
61. Matthys H, Erhardt J, Ruhle K. Objectivation of the effect of antitussive agents using tussometry in patients with chronic cough. Schweizerische Medizinische Wochenschrift 1985; 115: 307–311
62. Nespoli L, Monafo V, Bonetti F, Terraciano L, Savio G. Clinical evaluation of letosteine activity in the treatment of acute febrile bronchitis in children. Double blind controlled study versus placebo. Minerva Pediatrica 1989; 41: 515–520
63. Bergogne-Berezin E, Berthelot G, Kafe H, Dournovo P. Influence of fluidifying agent (bromhexine) on the penetration of antibiotics into respiratory secretions. International Journal of Clinical Pharmacology Research 1985; 5: 341–344
64. Petty T. The national mucolytic study: results of a randomised double blind placebo controlled study of iodinated glycerol in chronic obstructive bronchitis. Chest 1990; 97: 75–83
65. Barberi I, Macchia A, Spata N, Scaricabarozzi I, Nava M. Double blind evaluation of nimesulide vs lysine-aspirin in the treatment of paediatric acute respiratory tract infections. Drugs 1993; 46 (suppl 1): 219–221
66. Macfarlane JT, Holmes WF, Macfarlane RM, Lewis S. Reducing reconsultation for acute lower respiratory tract illness with an information leaflet: a randomised controlled study of patients in primary care. British Journal of General Practice 1997; 47: 719–722
67. Lea P. A double blind controlled evaluation of the nasal decongestant effect of Day Nurse(Reg.Trademark) in the common cold. Journal of International Medical Research 1984; 12(2): 124–127
68. Erffmeyer J, McKenna W, Lieberman P. Efficacy of phenyephrine-phenylpropanolamine in the treatment of rhinitis. Southern Medical Journal 1982; 75: 562–564
69. Akerlund A, Klint T, Olen L, Rundkrantz H. Nasal decongestant effect of oxymetazoline in the common cold: an objective dose response study in 106 patients. Journal of Laryngology and Otology 1989; 103: 743–746
70. Hayden F, Diamond L, Wood P, Korts D, Wecker M. Effectiveness and safety of intranasal ipratropium

bromide in common colds. A randomised double blind, placebo-controlled trial. Annals of Internal Medicine 1996; 125: 89–97

71. Bollag U, Albrecht E, Wingert W. Medicated versus saline nose drops in the management of upper respiratory infection. Helvetica Paediatrica Acta 1984; 39: 341–345

72. Adam P, Stiffman M, Blake R. A clinical trial of hypertonic saline nasal spray in subjects with the common cold or rhinosinusitis. Archives of Family Medicine 1998; 7: 39–43

73. Graf P, Juto E. Correlation between objective nasal mucosal swelling and estimated stuffiness during long term use of vasocontrictors. Journal of Otorhino-Laryngology its Related Specialties 1994; 56(6): 334–339

74. Thomas S, Clark K, Allen R, Smith S. A comparison of the cardiovascular effects of phenylpropanolamine and phenylephrine containing proprietary cold remedies. British Journal of Clinical Pharmacology 1991; 32(6): 705–711

75. Singh M. Heated, humidified air for the common cold. Cochrane Library, updated April 1999

76. Arroll B, Kenealy T. Antibiotics for the common cold. Cochrane Library, updated July 1998

77. Luks D, Anderson M. Antihistamines and the common cold: a review and critique of the literature. Journal of General Internal Medicine 1996; 11(4): 240–244

78. Marshall I. Zinc for the common cold. Cochrane Library, updated 1998

79. Melchart D, Linde K, Fischer P, Kaesmayr J. Echinacea for preventing and treating the common cold. Cochrane Library, updated October 1998

80. Barrow G, Higgins W, Al-Nakib. The effect of intranasal necrodomil sodium on viral upper respiratory tract infections in human volunteers. Clinical and Experimental Allergy 1990; 20: 45–51

81. Aberg N, Aberg B, Alestig K. The effect of inhaled and intranasal sodium cromoglycate on symptoms of upper respiratory tract infections. Clinical and Experimental Allergy 1996; 26: 1045–1050

82. Catalano G, Serra A, Salami A, Tinelli E. Effect of tiaprofenic acid on nasal mucociliary transport time. Acta Otorhinolaryngologica Italica 1990; 10(suppl 28): 63–72

83. Garibaldi R. Epidemiology of community aquired respiratory tract infections in adults: incidence aetiology and impact. American Journal of Medicine 1985; 78(S6b): 33–37

84. Wiselka M. Influenza: diagnosis management and prophylaxis. British Medical Journal 1994; 308: 1341–1345

85. Govaert T, Dinant G, Aretz K, Knotternus J. The predictive value of influenza symptomatology in elderly people. Family Practice 1998; 15: 16–22

86. Broggini M, Botta V, Benvenuti C. Flurbiprofen versus ASA in influenza symptomatology: a double blind study. International Journal of Clinical Pharmacology Research 1986; 6: 485–488

87. Bernasconi P, Massera E. Evaluation of a new form of nimesulide for the treatment of influenza. Drugs under Experimental and Clinical Research 1985; 11: 739–743

88. Jefferson T, Demicheli V, Deeks J, Rivetti D. Amantadine and Rimantadine for preventing and treating influenza A in adults. Cochrane Library, updated February 1998

89. Gross P, Hermogenes A, Sacks H, Lau J, Levandowski R. The efficacy of influenza vaccine in elderly persons: a meta-analysis and review of the literature. Annals of Internal Medicine 1995; 123: 518–527

90. Feibach N, Beckett W. Prevention of respiratory infections in adults. Archives of Internal Medicine 1999; 154: 2545–2557

91. Cates C, Jefferson T, Bara A. Vaccines for preventing influenza in people with asthma. Cochrane Library, updated July 1998

92. AHCPR. Evidence report/technology assessment number 9: Diagnosis and treatment of acute bacterial rhinosinusitis, 1999

93. Williams J, Simel D. Does this patient have sinusitis? Journal of the American Medical Association 1999; 270: 1242–1246

94. Williams J, Simel D, Roberts L, Samsa G. Clinical evaluation for sinusitis: making the diagnosis by history and physical examination. Annals of Internal Medicine 1992; 117: 705–710

95. Gwaltney J, Sydnor A, Sande M. Etiology and anti-microbial treatment of acute sinusitis. Annals of Otology, Rhinology and Laryngology 1981; suppl 90: 68–71

96. Lindbaek M, Kaastad E, Dolvik S, Johnsen U, Laerum E, Hjortdahl P. Antibiotic treatment of patients with mucosal thickening in the paranasal sinuses and validation of cut-off points in sinus CT. Rhinology 1998; 36: 7–11

97. Lindbaek M, Hjordtdahl P, Johnsen U. Use of symptoms signs and blood tests to diagnose acute sinus infections in primary care: comparison with computed tomography. Family Medicine 1996; 28: 183–188

98. Berg O, Carenfelt C. Analysis of symptoms and signs in the maxillary sinus empyema. Acta Otorhinolaryngologica (Stockholm) 1988; 105: 343–349

99. Williams J, Aguilar C, Makelar M, et al. Antimicrobial therapy for acute sinusitis. Cochrane Library, updated March 1999

100. Stalman W. The end of antibiotic treatment in adults with acute sinusitis-like complaints in general

practice? A placebo-controlled double blind randomised doxycycline trial. British Journal of General Practice 1997; 47: 794–799

101. Hansen J, Schmidt H, Grinsted P. A randomised double blind placebo controlled trial of penicillin V in the treatment of acute maxillary sinusitis in adults in general practice. Scandinavian Journal of Primary Health Care 2000; 18: 44–47

102. Norrelund N. Treatment of Sinusitis in general practice. A controlled investigation of pivampicillin (pondocillin). [Danish] Ugeskrift for Laeger. Voekr.Laeger 1978; 140: 2792–2795

103. Van Buchem F, Knotternus J, Schrinjnemaekers V, Peeters MF. Primary care based randomised placebo controlled trial of antibiotic treatment in acute maxillary sinusitis. Lancet 1997; 349: 683–687

104. Lindbaek M, Hjortdahl P, Johnsen U. Randomised, double blind, placebo controlled trial of penicillin V and amoxycillin in treatment of acute sinus infections in adults. British Medical Journal 1996; 313: 325–329

105. Wiklund L, Stierna P, Berglund R, Westrin K, Tonnesson M. The efficacy of oxymetazoline administered with a nasal bellows container and combined with oral phenoxymethylpenicillin in the treatment of acute maxillary sinusitis. Acta Oto-rhinolaryngologica (Stockholm) 1994; 515 (suppl): 57–64

106. McCormick D, John S, Swischuk L, Uchida T. A double blind placebo controlled trial of a decongestant antihistamine for the treatment of sinusitis in children. Clinical Pediatrics (Philadelphia) 1996; 35: 457–460

107. Braun J, Alabort J, Mochel F et al. Adjunct effect of loratidine in the treatment of acute sinusitis in patients with allergic rhinitis. Allergy 1997; 52: 650–655

108. Meltzer E, Orgel H, Backhaus J et al. Intranasal flunisolide spray as an adjunct to oral antibiotic therapy for sinusitis. Journal of Allergy and Clinical Immunology 1993; 92: 812–823

109. Darlan I, Erkan C, Dakir M, Derrak S, Baoaran M. Intranasal budesonide spray as an adjunct to oral antibiotic therapy for acute sinusitis in children. Annals of allergy asthma & immunology 1999; 78: 598–601

110. Tutkun A, Inanli S, Batman C, Uneri C, Sehitoglu M. The impact of intranasal steroid as an adjunct therapy for acute sinusitis. Marmara Medical Journal 1996; 9: 11–14

111. Frachet B, Genee N, Rezvani Y. Efficacy and tolerability of tiaprofenic acid in acute sinusitis in adults. Annales d Otoaryngologie et de Chirurgie Cervicofaciale (French) 1991; 108: 364–369

112. Bobin S, Ditisheim A, Le P, Harboun E, Avid N. A double blind placebo controlled trial of niflumic acid in the treatment of acute sinusitis. Current therapeutic research clinical & experimental 1989; 46: 1119–1128

113. Taub S. The use of bromelains in sinusitis: a double blind clinical evaluation. Eye ear nose & throat monthly 1967; 46: 361

114. Ryan R. A double blind clinical evaluation of bromelains in the treatment of acute sinusitis. Headache 1967; 7: 13–17

115. Seltzer A. Adjunctive use of bromelains in acute sinusitis: a controlled study. Eye ear nose & throat monthly 1967; 46: 1281–1288

116. Harris P. A comparison of bisolvomycin and oxytetracycline in the treatment of acute infective sinusitis. Practitioner 1971; 207: 814–817

117. Godley F. Chronic sinusitis: an update. American Family Physician 2000; 45(5): 2190–2199

118. Lazar R, Yuonis R, Parvey L. Comparison of plain radiographs, coronal CT, and intraoperative findings in children with chronic sinusitis. Otolaryngology – Head and Neck Surgery 1992; 107: 29–34

119. Otten H, Antvelink J, Ruyter-de-Wildt H, Rietema S, Siemelink R, Hordijk G. Is antibiotic treatment of chronic sinusitis effective in children. Clinical Otolaryngology 1994; 19: 215–217

120. Otten F. Conservative treatment of chronic maxillary sinusitis in children. Acta Otorhinolaryngologica Belgica 1997; 51: 173–175

121. Hashiba M. Clinical efficacy of long term macrolide therapy for chronic sinusitis – comparison between erythromycin and clarithromycin. Practica Otologica 1997; 90: 717–727

122. Legent F, Bordure P, Beauvillain C, Berche P. A double blind comparison of ciprofloxacin and amoxycillin clavulanate in the treatment of chronic sinusitis. Chemotherapy 1994; 40(suppl 1): 8–15

123. Qvarnberg Y, Kantola O, Salo J, Tiovanen M, Valtonen H, Vuori E. Influence of topical steroids treatment of maxillary sinusitis. Rhinology 1992; 30: 103–112

124. Sykes D, Wilson R, Chan K, Cole P. Relative importance of antibiotic and improved clearance in topical treatment of chronic muco-purulent rhinosinusitis. A controlled study. Lancet 1986; 2: 359–360

125. Schlenter W, Blessing R, Heintz B. Clinical efficacy of oral immunostimulant in adult patients with chronic purulent sinusitis. Laryngo-Rhino-Otologie (Stuttgart) 1989; 68: 671–674

126. Zagar S, Lofler-Badzek D. Broncho-Vaxom in children with chronic rhinosinusitis: a double blind clinical trial. J.Otorhinolaryngol Relat.Spec. 1988; 50: 397–404

▶ 17

Urinary tract infections

Paul Little

Importance

Urinary tract infections (UTIs) are among the most common bacterial infections seen by physicians. They are the most common bacterial infections occurring in women and second only to upper respiratory tract infections as a source of morbidity in children.

In children, vesico-ureteral reflux (VUR) of infected urine into the renal parenchyma (reflux nephropathy) can cause renal scarring. This can lead to poor renal growth, recurrent adult pyelonephritis, impaired glomerular filtration rate, early hypertension and end stage renal failure,[1-3] and renal hypertension and chronic renal failure in children.[4] Bacteriuria alone will not cause scarring but recurrent infection with VUR increases scarring.[1,5] It has been estimated that 80% of children younger than 5 years who have recurrent UTI and persistent VUR develop renal scarring.[6] Most scars develop before the age of 5 years,[7] although new scar formation does occur in older children with a diagnosis of probable pyelonephritis.[8,9] However, a review of all studies relating VUR to outcome questions the level of risk associated with VUR,[10] and most children with VUR do not develop high blood pressure.[11]

Review of evidence relating to indicator set

Screening

Children

In preschool children asymptomatic bacteriuria is rare (0.8% girls, negligible in boys),[12] screening results in a 20% false-positive rate, and there is no evidence that routine screening improves outcome.[13]

Pregnant women

In pregnancy 20–40% of women with asymptomatic bacteriuria develop pyelonephritis. A systematic review demonstrates that antibiotic treatment effectively clears bacteriuria and reduces the incidence of pyelonephritis, preterm delivery and low birthweight babies.[14] Whether short or long courses are required is unclear.[15]

Other groups

There is no accepted role for screening in otherwise healthy men and non-pregnant women.[16-18] There is controversy about screening in diabetics and the elderly since treatment of both groups has a high failure rate and a high rate of reinfection.[12]

Diagnosis

Children

Infants with a UTI may have malodorous urine, a changed urinary stream, or non-specific symptoms such as fever, irritability, failure to thrive or jaundice. For this reason children without an apparent source of fever should be evaluated for UTI.[19,20] Other symptoms suggesting UTI are secondary enuresis in older children or haematuria unrelated to trauma (indicator 3). School-age children have more 'classic' symptoms of UTI: dysuria, frequency, urgency and/or flank pain.

Adult women

In adults uncomplicated UTI is suggested by symptoms of bladder irritation (dysuria, frequency, nocturia, urgency) and occasionally haematuria. Upper tract infection is suggested by fever, rigors or back/flank pain.[21-24] Vaginal infections (Candida, Trichomonas) and urethritis (Chlamydia, Neisseria, herpes simplex virus) can also present with UTI-like symptoms.[22]

Other groups

Men with urethritis can also present with UTI-like symptoms (see above) (indicator 6.1). Those with acute prostatitis are often systemically unwell and have pelvic pain and/or a tender prostate. Chronic prostatitis and prostatic hypertrophy may be the underlying cause for recurrent UTI in men.

Urine culture in the diagnosis of UTI

Definitive diagnosis of UTI is by urine culture, but there is debate about the importance of making a definitive diagnosis in all groups, and debate as to the culture growth cut-offs to determine urine infection. Historically, 10^5 or more colony-forming units (cfu) per ml, usually with pyuria, was shown to differentiate between infection (often pyelonephritis) confirmed by bladder specimens of urine when compared to midstream urine (MSU).[25] More recently, young women presenting with symptomatic UTI were shown to have lower colony counts ($>10^2$ cfu/ml) not due to contamination[23] with a demonstrable response to treatment in controlled trials.[23,24] Half of those with low colony counts develop high colony counts within 2 days.[26] There have been similar findings of the validity of diagnosis of low colony counts in adult men[27] and in acute pyelonephritis.[28]

However, the practicality of using definitions of UTI based on low colony counts is still debated due to concerns about the laboratory findings and laboratory expertise in realistic clinical settings.[29] Furthermore, research on low colony counts is based on immediate and optimal laboratory facilities, whereas in the real clinical setting of primary care, specimens are often not stored immediately and not transported in refrigerated conditions, leading to delay in laboratory analysis. This is likely to inflate colony counts and result in more false-positive results. Most UK laboratories are not set up to report counts down to 10^2 cfu/ml, and 10^5 is the current Public Health Laboratory Service standard.

Urinalysis and dipsticks

Definitive diagnosis by urine culture can influence prognosis and treatment. Given the importance of confirming the diagnosis in children, and that urinalysis will miss 20% of infections (see below), a urine culture should always be done if UTI is suspected in children.

Considering specific tests in detail:

▶ *Nitrite and haematuria*: a nitrite test is not very sensitive, but reasonably specific,[23,29-31] and haematuria is similarly specific but not sensitive.[23,29,31]

▶ *Microscopy*: bacteriuria by microscopic examination is sensitive and specific compared to a standard diagnosis,[32] although a combination of bacteriuria, pyuria and a positive nitrite test probably performs better than any single test.[30] However, urine microscopy is impractical for most primary care physicians who have neither the time nor the expertise to perform microscopy.

▶ *Leucocyte esterase*: The leucocyte esterase test is moderately sensitive and specific, and combined with nitrite has sensitivity and specificity of approximately 80%,[33] but may be less sensitive for low colony counts.[34]

A systematic review of the use of dipsticks has highlighted the poor quality of the studies, and the lack of evidence from primary care.[31] In realistic clinical settings urinalysis may not perform well.[35]

Accurate diagnosis or empirical treatment for uncomplicated cases?

In one trial in adult women, the initial urine analysis or culture did not predict the response to treatment.[36] In a decision analytic model, obtaining an initial urine culture in all patients reduced expected symptom days by about 10% but increased expected cost by about 40%.[37]

Urine culture: situations where diagnosis is more important

Urine culture should be used both to confirm the diagnosis and guide therapy for patients at risk of either occult renal infection or 'complicated' UTI.[34,38-45] Complicated infections are found in the following circumstances:

▶ immunocompromised state

▶ suspected acute pyelonephritis

▶ structural or functional anomalies of the urinary tract

▶ pregnancy

▶ men

▶ recent instrumentation of the urinary tract.

Although there is no direct evidence that such a selective approach improves outcomes, the rationale for initial culture for 'complicated' infections is that if there is no quick response to therapy within 48 hours a rapid reappraisal based on the initial culture results is possible. This will ensure that there is maximal chance of eradicating the infection in groups who are already more unwell clinically or with a high risk of complications (indicator 2).

Treatment

The choice and duration of antibiotic treatment depends on the prognostic significance of infection in the particular group.

Treatment of uncomplicated UTI: antibiotics
Systematic reviews of treatment in women have shown that symptom duration is shorter with 7-day or longer courses compared to 3-day or single-dose treatment,[46,47] but side-effects of longer courses are much greater, including thrush and skin rash.[47] A decision analysis model comparing single-dose with 10-day courses found that single-dose treatments were more cost-effective because the 3- to 4-fold incidence of side-effects with longer courses outweighed the slightly better cure rates.[37] However, the side-effects of longer courses may be due to the use of trimethoprim-sulfamethoxazole in most trials. A single dose of trimethoprim alone cleared urine in 82% within 2 weeks, compared with 94% for 7 days in a larger trial[48] and there were no significant differences in adverse effects. A comparison of 3 days and 10 days of trimethoprim documented very similar rates of clearance (94% and 97% respectively)[24] (indicator 6).

Which antibiotic?
The combination of trimethoprim with sulphonamide has been shown to be no more effective than trimethoprim alone[49-52] and trimethoprim probably has a lower side-effect profile. Amoxycillin and nitrofurantoin have higher failure rates.[34,46,53,54] Although quinolones are effective[55,56] they should probably be reserved for patients with known resistance or allergy to other first-line agents, or where data from representative community samples suggest that resistance to trimethoprim is high. This would avoid unnecessary expense and the promotion of resistant strains[57] (indicator 5).

No treatment and other treatments
It has been reported that 50% of subjects with documented bacteriuria will settle both symptomatically and bacteriologically within 3 days, and thus the utility of any antibiotic treatment must be questioned in view of the side-effects.[58] This finding is supported by a small trial in general practice for women with symptomatic UTI and low colony counts where 76% of the cotrimoxazole-treated group and 60% of the placebo group were symptom-free by 4 days.[59]

Cranberry juice may reduce bacteriuria[60] and change urinary pH.[61] A systematic review documented that cranberry juice may prevent UTI,[62] although the evidence for treating symptomatic UTIs is limited.[63]

Treatment of pyelonephritis
Severe pyelonephritis with nausea and vomiting requires parenteral antibiotics, which in practical terms usually means initial hospitalisation. However, continuous

parenteral therapy is not mandatory.[64–66] Regarding duration, in one trial 2 weeks of antibiotics was as effective as 6 weeks, with symptoms and bacteriuria resolving by 7 days.[67] In another trial for hospitalised patients a 3-week course of antibiotics was more effective than a 1-week course[68] (indicators 4 and 7).

Treatment in children

Children with uncomplicated UTI can be treated on an outpatient basis with a 7- to 10-day course of a broad spectrum antibiotics. Shorter courses are associated with higher recurrence rates.[69] Observational studies suggest increased rates of renal scarring in children where the diagnosis and treatment are delayed.[70]

Preventing recurrence

Once-weekly perfloxacin is effective in preventing recurrence for women with recurrent UTIs.[71] In a large trial in patients with recurrent UTI compared with placebo (65% recurrence) there were lower rates with methenamine hippurate (34%), nitrofurantoin (25%) and trimethoprim (10%).[72] A smaller trial showed that recurrence was effectively prevented equally well with trimethoprim, cotrimoxazole or nitrofurantoin.[73] Two trials in children with documented UTI indicate that prophylactic antibiotics reduce the rate of recurrence.[74,75] Methenamine hippurate effectively prevented recurrence (73% fewer infections) in a small double-blind crossover study for patients with recurrent cystitis,[76] and in another small trial for patients with neurogenic bladder dysfunction.[77] For patients with spinal cord injury, low-dose daily cotrimoxazole is effective.[78]

Follow-up

There is no clear agreement about the necessity for follow-up urine cultures. There is evidence that providing routine follow-up for uncomplicated infection is not necessary.[36,79] There is no evidence that a routine reassessment is necessary, but a child not improving should probably be followed up carefully in view of the risk of complications (pyelonephritis, renal scarring, septicaemia) (indicator 8).

Investigation

Investigation in men

There is considerable uncertainty about the clinical and prognostic significance of abnormalities detected by investigation,[80–82] and many would not alter their therapeutic approach if abnormalities were present.[83,84] Prostatic infection accounts for the majority of relapse in men[85] which usually responds to a prolonged course of antibiotics. Thus there is no clear need to refer for investigation unless recurrent infections do not respond to a prolonged course of antibiotics.

Investigation in children

If the diagnosis of VUR is delayed beyond the age of 5, there is impaired renal growth, whereas if the diagnosis is made before age 5, 'catch-up' renal growth can occur,[86] and severity of scarring is significantly related to delay in diagnosis.[87] A cohort of UK children with a normal DMSA scan after their first UTI showed follow-up scarring in 1:40 (5/209) children aged 3 and none (0/220) of the children aged 4.[7] Thus the time of greatest risk from recurrent UTIs with VUR is likely to be up to the age of 4. After this, if initial DMSA scans are normal, the risk of new scarring is low (indicator 9).

Recommended quality indicators for urinary tract infection

Diagnosis
1 In men aged 15+ presenting with dysuria, enquiry should be made about a history of urethral discharge
2 Prior to antibiotic treatment, a urine culture should be obtained for patients who have dysuria and any 'complicating' factor (i.e. with complications or where complications are more likely):
   a. immunocompromised state
   b. suspected diagnosis of pyelonephritis
   c. structural/functional anomalies of urinary tract
   d. pregnancy
   e. men
   f. children
   g. recent instrumentation of the urinary tract
3 If an infant or child under the age of 12 presents with any of the following symptoms/signs (unless the child is admitted immediately to hospital), a urine culture should be performed:
   a. malodorous urine, abnormal urinary stream or change in urinary stream, or unexplained systemic symptoms (e.g. failure to thrive, jaundice, fever in a neonate)
   b. dysuria, frequency, urgency, flank pain (unrelated to trauma)
   c. haematuria unrelated to trauma
   d. secondary enuresis

Treatment
4 Patients diagnosed with an upper tract or other 'complicated' UTI should receive treatment with antimicrobials
5 Quinalones should not be used as the first line agents for patients with uncomplicated UTIs without justification
6 If uncomplicated lower tract infections are treated with antibiotics, treatment should not exceed 5 days
7 Patients should be prescribed antimicrobial therapy for at least 7 days for a suspected upper tract infection (pyelonephritis)
8 Children with suspected or confirmed UTI should be reassessed within 10 days
9 Children less than 5 years old with a first UTI should be referred for specialist opinion within 1 month.
10 Children aged 5–12 with suspected pyelonephritis who have not had urological investigation should be referred for specialist opinion

---

The effectiveness of routine diagnostic imaging is debatable,[70] and there is no clear consensus as to which children with UTIs require full radiological work-up.[6,8,88–90] However, children with VUR cannot be identified clinically,[91,92] Thus there is no clear alternative to investigation after the first UTI, and to providing prophylaxis until investigation is performed. Investigation should take account of the fact that although older children with pyelonephritis do develop renal scars, most scarring has occurred by the age of 5, and for children with no scarring by age 4 new scars are unlikely (indicator 10).

Antibiotic prophylaxis in children
Treatment of children with VUR and UTIs is likely to be effective in preventing recurrence of UTI as shown by two small trials of prophylaxis for children with recurrent UTI.[74,75]

Medical treatment or surgical treatment for VUR?
Recent trials and a meta-analysis of older trial data suggest little difference between surgical correction and medical management in terms of recurrent infection or scarring,[10,86,93,94] although more children with medical treatment may have pyelonephritis (21% versus 10% in the surgical group).[95]

Overview of data sources used in this review

This review is based on a search of Medline for reviews and trials for the years 1990–7 and a search of the Cochrane Library for systematic reviews and database of randomised controlled trials using the terms 'urinary tract infection' (UTI), 'urine and infections', 'cystitis and pyelonephritis'.

References

1. Berg U. Long term follow-up of renal morphology and function in children with recurrent pyelonephritis. Journal of Urology 1992; 148: 1715–1720
2. Martinell J, Claeson I, Lidin-Janson G, Jodal U. Urinary infection reflux and scarring in females continuously followed for 13–38 years. Pediatric Nephrology 1995; 9: 131–136
3. Jacobson S, Eklof O, Erikkson C, Lins L, Tidgren B. Development of hypertension and uraemia after pyelonephritis in childhood. British Medical Journal 1989; 299: 703–706
4. White R. Management of urinary tract infection and vesico-ureteric reflux in children. British Medical Journal 1990; 300: 1291–1292
5. Verrier-Jones K, Asscher A, Verrier-Jones E, Mattholie K, Leach K. Glomerular filtration rate in schoolgirls with covert bacteriuria. British Medical Journal 1982; 285: 1307–1310
6. Woodhead J. Genitourinary problems. In: Derschewitz R, ed. Ambulatory pediatric care. Philadelphia: Lippincott, 1993; 436–441
7. Vernon S, Coulthard M, Lambert H, Keir M, Matthews J. New renal scarring in children who at age 3 and 4 years had had normal scans with DMSA: follow-up study. British Medical Journal 1997; 315: 905–908
8. Andrich M, Majd M. Diagnostic imaging in the evaluation of first urinary tract infection in infants and young children. Pediatrics 1992; 90(3): 436–441
9. Benador D, Benador N, Slosman D, Mermillod B, Girardin E. Are younger children at highest risk of renal sequelae after pyelonephritis. Lancet 1997; 349: 17–19
10. Shanon A, Feldman W. Methodological limitations in the literature on vesico-ureteric reflux: a critical review. Journal of Pediatrics 1990; 117(2): 171–178
11. Wolfish N, Delbrouck N, Shanon A, Matzinger M, Stenstrom R, McLaine P. Prevalence of hypertension in children with primary vesicoureteric reflux. Journal of Pediatrics 1993; 123(4): 559–563
12. Zhanel G, Harding G, Guay D. Asymptomatic bacteriuria. Archives of Internal Medicine 1990; 150: 1389–1396
13. Kemper K, Avner E. The case against screening urinanalysis for asymptomatic bacteriuria in children. American Journal of Diseases of Children 1992; 146: 343–346
14. Smaill F. Antibiotics for asymptomatic bacteriuria in pregnancy. Cochrane Library, updated 1996
15. Villar J, Lydon-Rochelle M, Gulmezoglu A. Duration of treatment for asymptomatic bacteriuria during pregnancy. Cochrane Library 1997, updated October 1997

16. Pels R, Bor D, Woolhandler S, Himmelstein D, Lawrence R. Dipstick urinanalysis of asymptomatic adults for urinary tract disorders. Journal of the American Medical Association 1989; 262(9): 1221–1224

17. Childs S, Egan R. Bacteriuria and urinary infections in the elderly. Urologic Clinics of North America 1996; 23(1): 43–54

18. Baladassarre J, Kaye D. Special problems of urinary tract infection in the elderly. Medical Clinics of North America 1991; 75: 375–390

19. Stull T, LiPuma J. Epidemiology and natural history of urinary tract infections in children. Medical Clinics of North America 1991; 75(2): 287–297

20. Lebel M. Urinary tract infections. In: Oski F, DeAngelis R, Feigin R, eds. Principles and practice of paediatrics. Philadelphia: Lippincott, 1994: 532–533

21. Dobbs FF, Fleming DM. A simple scoring system for evaluating symptoms, history and urine dipstick testing in the diagnosis of urinary tract infection. Journal of the Royal College of General Practitioners 1987; 37 : 100–104

22. Komaroff A. Acute dysuria in women. In: Panzer R, Black E, Griner P, eds. Diagnostic strategies for common medical problems. Philadelphia: American College of Physicians, 1991: 239–248

23. Stamm W, Counts G, Running K, Fihn S, Turck M, Holmes K. Diagnosis of coliform infections in acutely dysuric women. New England Journal of Medicine 1982; 307: 463–468

24. Gossius G, Vorland L. The treatment of acute dysuria-frequency syndrome in adult women: double blind randomized comparison of three day versus ten day trimethoprim therapy. Current therapeutic research clinical & experimental 1985; 37: 34–42

25. Kass E. Bacteriuria and the diagnosis of infections of the urinary tract. Archives of Internal Medicine 1957; 100: 709

26. Arav-Bolger R, Leibovici L, Danon Y. Urinary tract infections with low colony counts and high colony counts in young women: spontaneous remission. Archives of Internal Medicine 1994; 154: 300–304

27. Lipsky B, Ireton R, Fihn S, Hackett R, Berger R. Diagnosis of bacteriuria in men: specimen collection and culture interpretation. Journal of Infectious Diseases 1987; 155: 847–854

28. Bollgren I, Engstrom C, Hammarlind M, Kallenius G, Ringertz H, Svenson S. Low urinary counts of P-fimbriated E. coli in presumed acute pyelonephritis. Archives of Disease in Childhood 1984; 59: 102–106

29. Pappas P. Laboratory in the diagnosis and management of UTI. Medical Clinics of North America 1991; 75(2): 313–325

30. Bailey B. Urinanalysis predictive of urine culture results. Journal of Family Practice 1995; 40(1): 45–50

31. Moore RA, Hawke C, Newall R, Price C, Deeks J, Warner G. Reagent dipsticks and urinary tract infection in general practice: a systematic review from published data. Unpublished, 1998

32. Jenkins R, Fenn J, Matsen J. Review of urine microscopy for bacteriuria. Journal of the American Medical Association 1986; 255: 3397

33. Pfaller M, Koontz F. Laboratory evaluation of leucocyte esterase and nitrite tests for the detection of bacteriuria. Journal of Clinical Microbiology 1985; 21(5): 840–842

34. Johnson J, Stamm W. Urinary tract infections in women: diagnosis and treatment. Annals of Internal Medicine 1989; 111(11): 906–917

35. Winkens RA, Leffers P, Trienekens TA, Stobberingh EE. The validity of urine examination for urinary tract infections in daily practice. Family Practice 1995; 12(3): 290–293

36. Schulz H, McCaffrey T, Keys T, Nobrega F. Acute cystitis: a prospective study of laboratory tests and duration of therapy. Mayo Clinic Proceedings 1984; 59: 391–397

37. Carlson A, Mulley A. Management of acute dysuria. Annals of Internal Medicine 1985; 102: 244–249

38. Komaroff A. Urinalysis and urine culture in women with dysuria. Annals of Internal Medicine 1986; 104: 212–218

39. Rubin R, Fang S, Jones S. Single dose amoxycillin for urinary tract infection: multicenter trial using antibody coated bacteria localization technique. Journal of the American Medical Association 1980; 244 : 561–564

40. Cardenas J, Quinn E, Rokker G, Bavinger J, Pohlod D. Single dose cephalexin therapy for acute bacterial urinary tract infections and acute urethral syndrome with bladder bacteriuria. Antimicrobial Agents and Chemotherapy 1986; 29: 383–385

41. Cattell W. Urinary tract infections in adults. Postgraduate Medical Journal 1985; 61: 907–913

42. Anderson R. Urinary tract infections in compromised hosts. Urologic Clinics of North America 1986; 13: 727–734

43. Preheim L. Complicated urinary tract infections. American Journal of Medicine 1985; 79(2A): 62–66

44. Forland M, Thomas V, Shelokov A. Urinary tract infections in patients with diabetes mellitus. Journal of the American Medical Association 1977; 238: 1924–1926

45. Schardijn G, Statius-van-Eps L, Pauw W, Hoefnagel C, Nooyen W. Comparison of reliability of tests to distinguish upper from lower urinary tract infection. British Medical Journal 1984; 289: 284–287

46. Norrby S. Short term treatment of uncomplicated lower urinary tract infection in women. 1990; 12 (3): 458–467

47. Leibovicki L, Wysenbeek A. Single Dose antibiotic treatment for symptomatic urinary tract infections in women: a meta-analysis of randomised trials. Quarterly Journal of Medicine 1991; 285: 43–57

48. Osterberg E, Aberg H, Hallander H, Kallner A, Lundin A. Efficacy of single dose versus seven day trimethoprim treatment of cystitis in women. Journal of Infectious Diseases 1990; 161: 942–947

49. Brumfitt W, Pursell R. Double blind trial to compare ampicillin, cephalexin, co-trimazole, and trimethoprim in the treatment of UTI. British Medical Journal 1972; 2: 673–676

50. Harbord R, Gruneberg R. Treatment of urinary tract infection with single dose of amoxycillin, co-trimoxazole, or trimethoprim. British Medical Journal 1981; 283: 1301–1302

51. Mabeck C, Vejlsgaard R. Treatment of urinary tract infections with sulphonamide and/or trimethoprim. A preliminary report from a multipractice study. Infection 1979; 7(suppl 4): s414–s415

52. Keenan T, Eliott J, Bishop V, Peddie B, Bailey R. Comparison of trimethoprim alone with cotrimoxazole and sulphamethiazole for the treatment of urinary tract infections. New Zealand Medical Journal 2000; 96: 341–342

53. Stamm W, Hooton T. Management of urinary tract infections in adults. New England Journal of Medicine 1993; 329: 1328–1334

54. Elder N. Acute urinary tract infection in women. Postgraduate Medicine 1992; 92: 159–172

55. Stein G, Mummaw N, Goldstein E. A multicenter comparative trial of three day norfloxacin vs ten day sulphamethoxazole and trimethoprim for the treatment of uncomplicated urinary tract infections. Archives of Internal Medicine 1987; 147: 1760–1762

56. Hooton T, Johnson C, Winter C, Kuwarmura L, Robers M, Roberts P. Single and three day regimes of ofloxacin vs trimethoprim-sulphamethoxazole for acute cystitis in women. Antimicrobial Agents and Chemotherapy 1991; 35(7): 1479–1483

57. Sable C, Scheld W. Fluoroquinolones: how to use (but not over use) these antibiotics. Geriatrics 1993; 48: 41–51

58. Brumfitt W, Hamilton-Miller J. Consensus viewpoint on the management of urinary infections. Journal of Antimicrobial Chemotherapy 1994; 33 (suppl A): 147–153

59. Brooks D, Garrett G, Hollihead R. Sulphadimidine, co-trimoxazole and a placebo in the management of symptomatic urinary tract infection in general practice. Journal of the Royal College of General Practitioners 1972; 22: 695–703

60. Avorn J, Monane M. Reduction of bacteriuria and pyuria after ingestion of cranberry juice. Journal of the American Medical Association 1994; 271: 751–754

61. Kinney A, Blount M. Effect of cranberry juice on urinary pH. Nursing Research 1979; 28: 287–290

62. Jepson R, Mihaljevic L, Craig J. Cranberries for preventing urinary tract infections. Cochrane Library, updated 1998

63. Jepson R, Mihaljevic L, Craig J. Cranberries for treating urinary tract infections. Cochrane Library, updated 1998

64. Wing D, Hendershott C, Debuque L, Millar L. A randomised trial of three antibiotic regimens for the treatment of pyelonephritis in pregnancy. Obstetrics and Gynecology 1998; 92: 249–253

65. Millar L, Wing D, Paul R, Grimes D. Outpatient treatment of pyelonephritis in pregnancy: a randomised controlled trial. Obstetrics and Gynecology 1995; 86: 560–564

66. Angel J, O'Brien W, Finan M, Morales W, Lake M, Knuppel R. Acute pyelonephritis in pregnancy: a prospective study of oral versus intravenous antibiotic therapy. Obstetrics and Gynecology 1990; 76: 28–32

67. Stamm W, McKevitt M, Counts G. Acute renal infection in women: treatment with trimethoprim-sulphamethoxazole or ampicillin for two or six weeks. Annals of Internal Medicine 1987; 106: 341–345

68. Jernelius H, Zbornik J, Bauer C. One or three week treatment of acute pyelonephritis. A double blind comparison using a fixed combination of pivampicillin plus pivmecillinam. Acta Medica Scandinavica 1988; 223: 469–477

69. Moffatt M, Embree J, Grimm P, Law B. Short course antibiotic therapy for urinary tract infections in children: a methodological review of the literature. American Journal of Diseases of Children 1988; 142: 57–61

70. Dick P, Feldman W. Routine diagnostic imaging for childhood urinary tract infections: a systematic overview. Journal of Pediatrics 1996; 128: 15–22

71. Guibert J, Humbert G, Meyrier A et al. Antibioprophylaxis for recurrent cystitis. a randomised double blind trial with two perfloxacin regimes. Presse Medicale 1995; 24: 213–216

72. Kasanen A, Junnila S, Kaarsalo E, Hajba A, Sundquist H. Secondary prevention of recurrent urinary tract infections. Comparison of the effect of placebo, methenamine hippurate, nitrofurantoin, and trimethoprim alone. Scandinavian Journal of Infectious Diseases 1982; 14: 293–296

73. Stamm W, Counts G, Wagner K et al. Antimicrobial prophylaxis of recurrent urinary tract infections: a double-blind, placebo-controlled trial. Annals of Internal Medicine 1980; 92: 770–775

74. Smellie J, Katz G, Gruneberg R. Controlled trial of prophylactic treatment in childhood urinary tract infection. Lancet 1978; ii: 175–178

75. Lohr J, Nunley D, Howards S, Ford R. Prevention of recurrent urinary tract infections in girls. Pediatrics 1977; 59: 562–565

76. Cronberg S, Welin C, Henriksson L, Hellten S, Persson K, Stenberg P. Prevention of recurrent acute cystitis by methenamine hippurate: double blind crossover long term study. British Medical Journal 1987; 294: 1507–1508

77. Kevorkian C, Merritt J, Ilstrup D. Methenamine mandelate with acidification: an effective urinary antiseptic in patients with neurogenic bladder. Mayo Clinic Proceedings 1984; 59: 523–529

78. Gribble M, Puterman M. Prophylaxis of urinary tract infection in persons with recent spinal injury: A prospective randomised double blind, placebo controlled study of trimethoprim-sulphamethoxazole. American Journal of Medicine 1993; 95: 141–152

79. Winickoff R, Wilner S, Gall G, Laage T, Barnett G. Urine culture after the treatment of uncomplicated cystitis in women. Southern Medical Journal 1981; 74(2): 165–169

80. Donker P, Kakiailatu F. Preoperative evaluation of patients with bladder outlet obstruction with particular regard to excretory urography. Transactions of the American Association of Genito–Urinary Surgeons 1978; 69: 44–45

81. Christofferson I, Moller I. Excretory urography: a superfluous routine examination in patients with prostatic hypertrophy. European Urology 1981; 7: 65–67

82. Krieger J. Prostatitis syndromes: pathophysiology, differential diagnosis and treatment. Sexually Transmitted Diseases 1984; 11: 100–112

83. Lipsky B. Urinary tract infections in men. Annals of Internal Medicine 1989; 110: 138–150

84. Corrado M, Grad C, Sabbaj J. Norfloxacin in the treatment of urinary tract infections in men with and without identifiable urologic complications. American Journal of Medicine 1987; 82(suppl 6b): 70–74

85. Goroll A, Lawrence A, Melley A. Primary care medicine: office evaluation and management of the adult patient. Philadelphia: Lippincott, 1995

86. Birmingham Reflux Study Group. Prospective trial of operative versus non-operative treatment of severe vesico-ureteric reflux in children: five year observation. British Medical Journal 1987; 295: 237–241

87. Smellie J, Poulton A, Prescod N. Retrospective study of children with renal scarring associated with reflux and urinary infection. British Medical Journal 1994; 308: 1193–1198

88. Sherbotie J, Cornfield D. Management of urinary tract infections in children. Medical Clinics of North America 1991; 75(2): 287–297

89. Royal College of Physicians Working Group. Report of a working group of the research unit, Royal College of Physicians. Guidelines for the management of acute urinary tract infection in childhood. Journal of the Royal College of Physicians of London 1991; 25: 36–42

90. Pilling D, Postlethwaite R. Imaging in urinary tract infection. British Paediatric Association Standing Committee, 1996: CO/96/03

91. Smellie J, Normand I, Katz G. Children with urinary infection: a comparison of those with and without vesico-ureteric reflux. Kidney International 1981; 20: 717–722

92. Majd M, Rushton H, Jantausch B, Wiedermann B. Relationship among vesico-ureteric reflux, P-fimbriated E. coli, and acute pyelonephritis in children with febrile acute urinary tract infections. Journal of Pediatrics 1991; 119: 578–585

93. Smellie J. Management of children with severe vesico-ureteric reflux. Journal of Urology 1992; 148(5): 1676–1678

94. Weiss R, Duckett J, Spitzer A. Results of a randomised trial of medical versus surgical management of infants with grade III and grade IV primary VUR. The international reflux study in children. Journal of Urology 1992; 148(5): 1667–1673

95. Jodal U, Koskimies O, Hanson E et al. Infection pattern in children with vesico-ureteric reflux randomly allocated to operation or long term prophylaxis. Journal of Urology 1992; 148: 1650–1652

▶18

Cervical screening

Sue Wilson

Importance

Incidence, mortality and survival

Each year there are approximately 3400 new cases of cervical cancer diagnosed in England and Wales, and about 1200 deaths attributable to the disease.[1,2] An average GP will see a woman with a new diagnosis of cervical cancer every 4 years and 1 death attributable to cervical cancer every 10 years. Cervical cancer is not common but many more women have cervical changes that are not invasive (Table 18.1).

The 5-year survival rate for women diagnosed with cervical cancer is approximately 55%[4] and has remained relatively constant over time.[5] Survival is significantly associated with stage at diagnosis, ranging from 7% for advanced disease to 80% for women with early localised cancer.[6] The marked difference in survival provides an incentive to detect disease at an early stage when treatment is likely to be successful.

The natural history of the disease

The natural history of cervical carcinoma is not well understood. Preinvasive disease is most frequently diagnosed in women aged 25–44 years; invasive carcinoma and deaths occur most frequently in women aged over 60 years. It is, however, difficult to infer the natural history of the disease because:

▶ the identification of preclinical disease depends on the intensity of screening – it is likely that more cervical intraepithelial neoplasia (CIN) will be identified in those women who are more extensively screened

Table 18.1   Cervical screening programme: test results

Test result	Number of smears	Percent
Negative	3 290 581	83.6
Borderline changes	148 003	3.8
Mild dyskaryosis	83 635	2.1
Moderate dyskaryosis	29 529	0.7
Severe dyskaryosis	18 457	0.5
Suspected invasive carcinoma	1041	0.0
? Glandular neoplasia	2628	0.1
Inadequate	364 116	9.2
Total	3 937 990	

Source: Cervical Screening Programme, England 1998–99[3]

▶ the natural history of cervical carcinoma is affected by preclinical identification and treatment.

Evidence for effectiveness of screening

A randomised controlled study of cervical screening has never been undertaken. Evidence for the effectiveness of screening programmes is, therefore, based on observational studies showing decreases in cervical cancer mortality following the introduction of screening programmes.[6-8] In Britain the national call–recall scheme was not introduced until 1988.[9] During the period 1965–82 the decline in mortality from cervical cancer was 21% and since 1988 the mortality has fallen by 35%.[10] Modelling age and birth cohort effects suggests that screening may have reduced the death rate by up to 50%.[11]

The role of primary care

Primary care teams are well placed to provide a focus for cancer prevention activities as 75% of the population consult their GP at least once a year and during any 3-year period over 90% will have attended the practice.[12] Over 90% of the 4.4 million smears taken each year occur in primary care.[3] Primary care is responsible for a number of activities relating to cervical screening; these include process (e.g. taking smears, dealing with smear results and running an effective failsafe system), evaluation (e.g. assessing reasons for non-attendance, auditing inadequate smear rates) and more general issues such as providing information or reducing anxiety.[13,14]

Review of evidence relating to indicator set

Screening and diagnosis

The screening test

Cervical cytology is a screening tool that aims to detect asymptomatic precancerous conditions of the cervix.[15] Any clinical suspicion of cervical cancer is an indication for a referral and not for a cervical smear.[16] A proportion of CIN 3 may regress; however, as the risk of invasion is high[17] women with this condition are generally treated.[15] Severe dysplasia is a recognisable precursor of cervical cancer.[18] Large proportions of low-grade lesions (mild dyskaryosis or CIN 1) spontaneously regress and are usually managed by surveillance as long as the patient is expected to attend for follow-up.[19] The vast majority of smears that are taken are negative.[3]

The screening test involves visualising the cervix and collecting exfoliated cells by rotating a spatula twice over the surface. There are, however, difficulties with this test:[20]

▶ Small lesions may fail to exfoliate sufficient abnormal cells.[21]

▶ Adequacy of the sample is dependent on the presence of metaplastic and columnar cells of endocervical origin.[22,23]

▶ Adequacy of smears is operator and instrument dependent.[23-26]

▶ Recognition and grading of cell samples may vary between cytologists and over time.[27,28]

Smear tests tend to underestimate the presence of disease.[29-32] Fifty percent of invasive cancers arise in women who have been adequately screened.[33] False-negative rates may be related to the adequacy of sampling exfoliated cells which may in turn be dependent on operator expertise, the sampling device used or laboratory errors. The positive predictive value of a smear is low; only 1% of all referrals are cancerous and 43% found to be CIN 2, CIN 3 or adenocarcinoma in situ.[3] Less than half of all women referred have a condition requiring treatment.

What device should be used for cervical sampling?

It is important that the transformation zone is sampled.[34] This requires both appropriate training and the use of an appropriately shaped device.[23,35] Dyskaryosis is more likely to be detected in smears that contain endocervical cells,[23] and glandular atypia (precursor of adenocarcinoma in situ) can only be identified if endocervical cells are present.[36] Extended-tip spatulas are better devices than the Ayre spatula[23,24] and although they are more expensive, repetition of inadequate smears increases the cost of screening and generates anxiety.[23] If the transformation zone is not visible then sampling with an endocervical brush as well as ectocervical sampling may be necessary.[34]

Monitoring coverage

Coverage, or the level of compliance with a screening programme, is often used as an indicator of its success.[37] Compliance is defined as the proportion of the target population that receives the screening test. Compliance is a proxy for the real screening objective: to reduce mortality. The coverage of the target population (25–64 years) in England has been estimated to be in excess of 80% since 1992.[3] Coverage rates are related to deprivation levels and vary by health authority.

All screening programmes tend to have preferential uptake from the non-manual classes.[38] However, the incidence of cervical cancer is higher in manual groups.[39] It is therefore possible that increasing compliance in this group might be associated with an increased rate of case detection and a consequent increase in health gain.[40] It has been estimated that, with a screening interval of 3 years, increasing compliance from 70% to 80% reduces the incidence of cervical cancer from 2.1 to 1.6 per 10 000 women aged over 18 years.[41] However, attempts to increase the uptake of screening need to be conducted alongside initiatives to increase informed uptake.[42]

Which populations should be screened?

Defining low-risk women, whose probability of developing this disease is extremely remote, and discharging them from further screening should not only result in reassurance for the individual women but also generate significant cost savings for the screening programme as a whole.

Only 7 of the 1219 deaths that occurred in England and Wales in 1997 were in women aged under 25.[2] There is no evidence to support taking a smear in immunocompetent women under the age of 20.[15] Non-negative smears in teenagers may result from normal developmental changes; referral of such cases to colposcopy will generate anxiety for little or no benefit.[15]

Current guidelines are that screening should continue to age 65;[15] however, defining the appropriate upper age group for screening is difficult.[43] Almost maximal effectiveness is achieved by organised programmes with high coverage that initiate screening at 25 and continue with 3- to 5-yearly screening until the age of 60.[44] Smear test results demonstrating severe dyskaryosis or worse are more common in younger women (1.2% for women aged 25–29, 0.4% in women aged 50–64).[3] The incidence of CIN in women over the age of 50 who have been regularly screened is exceptionally low (18 000 smear tests to detect one new case of CIN 3)[43] (indicator 4).

There have been proposals for women at increased risk of cervical cancer to be targeted to improve the effectiveness of screening.[46] However, the high-risk groups (educational level, smoking status, oral contraceptive use, number of sexual partners)[9,34,47,48] are not routinely identifiable on a population basis and the resulting stigmatisation would be socially unacceptable.[10]

The rate of progression of the disease and the sensitivity of the screening test are the only two factors that should determine the optimal screening frequency.[49,50] A person's risk of getting the disease should not determine how frequently she is screened. The incidence of disease does, however, affect cost-effectiveness. Given that those at highest risk of cervical cancer are often the least compliant with screening, more intensive efforts are required to include these women in the screening programme. Since there is no reason to believe that the rate of progression is greater in these high-risk groups or that the test is less sensitive there is no reason to screen them more frequently[49] (indicator 3).

At what interval should screening occur?

Screening should occur at sufficiently frequent intervals to detect abnormal cytology during the detectable preclinical phase. Data from several cervical cancer screening programmes have been pooled to assess the optimum frequency of screening.[27] These data suggest that the incidence of cervical cancer can be reduced by 64% with a screening interval of 10 years, by 84% with a 5-year interval, and by 91%, 93% and 94% with intervals of 3, 2 and 1 years respectively. Annual or 2-yearly screening may produce only a minimally lower risk of invasive disease than screening every 3 years.[35] Modelling suggests that 5-yearly screening of women aged over 35 is the most cost-effective option.[51,52]

The Department of Health recommends that a smear should be taken at least every 5 years. The rate of interval cancers is higher in women with an interval of more than 3.5 years between smears compared with an interval of less than 3.5 years (relative risk 2.2, 95% CI 1.3–3.8) suggesting that the 5-year interval may be too long.[53] However, the cost-effectiveness of reducing the screening interval from 5 to 3 years has been questioned.[54–56] Improving coverage, call and recall, diagnostic accuracy and the follow-up of abnormal smears may be more cost-effective ways of improving the screening programme than reducing the screening interval.[55] There is little evidence to suggest that age is appreciably related to the sensitivity of screening or the sojourn time[50,57] and the practice of taking a second smear 1 year after the first ever smear has not been shown to be effective[58] (indicators 2 and 3).

Treatment and follow-up

What is the appropriate management of women with abnormal screening tests?

Reducing cancer mortality requires adequate follow-up and treatment of women who have positive screening tests. The natural history and management of mild dyskaryosis is controversial. Follow-up of such women suggests that up to 26–35% will progress to CIN 3 in 2 years although the majority regress.[19,59–61] The psychological sequelae of referral for colposcopy and treatment may be greater than the risk of serious disease.[62] Mild dyskaryosis is common and has a variable outcome; cytologists' recommendations are based pragmatically on local availability of services and vary from immediate colposcopy to a repeat smear. All women with persistent disease should be referred for colposcopy. Colposcopy should be considered the first time a women has a mildly dyskaryotic smear if it is unlikely that she will comply with cytological follow-up or if the smear is after conservative treatment for CIN (indicators 7 and 8).

The appropriate interval when women reported to have moderate dyskaryosis should be rescreened is less easy to establish. However, since cytology tends to underestimate the severity of disease, all cases of moderate dyskaryosis are usually referred for colposcopy although the scarcity of resources in some areas requires that referral is only for persistent disease.[63] There is agreement that severe dysplasia on cytology requires referral for diagnosis and treatment[15] and that referral should be immediate when cervical cancer is suspected (indicators 5 and 6).

Running an effective failsafe system

To reduce anxiety and improve the quality of care the practice should take responsibility for notifying all women of the result of smears performed within the practice.[64–66] The follow-up of women who have positive test results is the responsibility of the doctor who takes the smear[9] or is responsible for requesting that the smear be taken. This responsibility remains in place even though clinical care may be referred elsewhere.[58]

In practice the most effective means of running follow-up systems is for the computerised cytology laboratory to issue reminders where they have recommended a repeat smear or referral to colposcopy, but where no sample has been received. However, given that the responsibility lies with the practitioner it is recommended that primary care teams have their own systems in place (indicator 1).

Women have the right to refuse services;[67] however, it is important that there is clear protocol for terminating the responsibility of the smear taker. Women may refuse services for a variety of reasons including fear or ignorance. There is a responsibility on practitioners to ensure that women are informed about the risks and benefits of screening[68] before they cover themselves medicolegally by asking a patient to sign a form confirming her decision and keeping this with her medical records.

Evaluating the screening programme

The cytology laboratory provides the proportion of inadequate smears on a practice basis. However, although interpractice variation is important, appropriate audits will also assess inadequate rates by smear taker. This may be useful in identifying training needs.

Conclusion

In summary, cervical screening is safe and observational evidence suggests that organised screening programmes are associated with reductions in incidence and mortality. However, cervical cancer is a relatively rare disease, its natural history is not well understood and the Pap smear has low sensitivity which results in many women being investigated and treated unnecessarily.[69] Furthermore, many tests are technically unsatisfactory and have to be repeated, which may cause distress and anxiety to patients. The annual cost of this screening programme has been estimated as £132 million,[70] about 4 times the cost of the breast screening programme.[10]

High-level performance indicators that have been accepted by the NHS comprise incidence and mortality rates and age-standardised 5-year survival rates.[71] Such indicators are not suitable for primary care as the number of incident cases occurring within a practice population is too small.[72] The one high-level performance indicator that can be calculated at practice level is screening coverage. However, given the dearth of good-quality evidence confirming the value of screening, the appropriate population to be screened or the appropriate screening interval there must be caution in recommending the routine introduction of indicators aiming to improve compliance.

Recommended quality indicators for cervical screening

Screening

1 The medical record should contain the date and result of the last smear taken (for women aged 25–64 years)

2 Women should be offered routine screening no less frequently than 5-yearly (unless never sexually active with men or have had a hysterectomy for benign indications) unless refusal is documented

3 Women should be offered routine screening no more frequently than 3-yearly (unless the previous smear was anything other than negative or they are immunodeficient)

4 Women aged over 65 years should not be offered screening unless they have had 2 abnormal smears in the previous 5 years

Treatment

5 Women with history of cervical dysplasia should have had a smear performed within 12 months following the abnormal smear

6 Women with a severely abnormal smear should be referred by the GP for colposcopy within 2 weeks of the receipt of result

7 Women with a low-grade lesion should have either a repeat smear or colposcopy within 6 months

8 Women with borderline changes on their smear results who have had the abnormality documented on 3 consecutive smears should be offered referral for colposcopy

---

Overview of data sources used in this review

This review is based on the NHS Cervical Screening Programme Guidelines[15] and a primary care-based review of screening.[20] These sources were supplemented by a Medline search of English language literature (1990–2000) using the search terms 'cervix dysplasia' and 'cervix neoplasms' in conjunction with 'screening'. Additional electronic databases searched include the Cochrane Controlled Trials Register, the NHS Centre for Reviews and Dissemination database of reviews of effectiveness (DARE) and the Department of Health website.

Acknowledgements

This review has benefited considerably from the constructive comments provided by Cath Finn, Sally Warmington, Kate Thomas and Lesley Roberts; the differing perspectives of general practitioners, gynaecologists, health service researchers and lay persons has been extremely useful. Particular thanks are due to Helen Lester who has provided considerable support and detailed comments on early drafts. Emma Morrish of the West Midlands Cancer Intelligence Unit collated the national incidence and mortality data and Richard Winder of the NHSCSR provided many useful references.

References

1. Cancer Statistics: registrations 1992. Office for National Statistics. Series MBI, No. 25, 1998
2. Cancer 1971–97 CD-Rom. Office of National Statistics, 1999
3. Department of Health. Cervical Screening Programme, England: 1998–99. Department of Health Bulletin 1999/32. London: Department of Health, 1999
4. Monitor: Population and Health. Imperial Cancer Research Fund, Office of National Statistics MB1 98/1 London 1998
5. Wilson S, Woodman C. Costs and benefits of cervical screening. In: Luesley D, Jordan J, Richart RM, eds. Intraepithelial neoplasia of the lower genital tract. New York: Churchill Livingstone, 1995: 61–70
6. Cancer Research Campaign. Cancer of the cervix uteri. Factsheet 12.2, 1994
7. Laara E, Day NE, Hakama M. Trends in mortality from cancer in the Nordic countries: association with organised screening programmes. Lancet 1987; i: 1247–1249
8. Hakama M, Magnus K, Pettersson F, Storm H, Tulinius H. Effect of organised screening on the risk of cervical cancer in the Nordic countries. In: Miller AB, Chamberlain J, Day NE, Hakama M, Prorock PC, eds. Cancer screening. Cambridge: International Union Against Cancer, Cambridge University Press, 1991: 153–162
9. Department of Health and Social Security. Health service management: cervical cancer screening (Health circular HC(88)1). DHSS, 1988
10. Quinn MJ, Babb PJ, Jones J, Allen E. Effect of screening on the incidence of and mortality from cancer of the cervix in England: evaluation based on routinely collected statistics. British Medical Journal 1999; 318: 904–908
11. Sasieni P, Adams J. Effect of screening on cervical cancer mortality in England and Wales: analysis of trends with an age period cohort model. British Medical Journal 1999; 318: 1244–1245
12. Fallowfield LJ, Rodway A, Maum M. What are the psychological factors influencing attendance, non-attendance and re-attendance at a breast screening centre. Journal of the Royal Society of Medicine 1990; 83: 547–551
13. Austoker J. Cervical screening in primary care: guidelines for working with primary care. Oxford: NHSCSP, 1990
14. Austoker J. Cancer prevention in primary care: screening for cervical cancer. British Medical Journal 1994; 309: 241–248
15. Duncan ID. Guidelines for clinical practice and programme management NHSCSP publication no. 8. Sheffield: NHS Cervical Screening Programme, 1997

16. Department of Health. Referral guidelines for suspected cancer – consultation document. London: Department of Health, 1999

17. McIndoe WA, McLean MR, Jones RW, Mullins P. The invasive potential of carcinoma in situ of the cervix. Obstetrics and Gynecology 1984; 64(4): 451–458

18. Evans DJD, Hudson EA, Brown CL et al. Terminology in gynaecological cytopatholgy: report of the working party of the British Society for Clinical Cytology. Journal of Clinical Pathology 1986; 39: 933–944

19. Nasiell K, Roger V, Nasiell M. Behaviour of mild cervical dysplasia during long-term follow-up. Obstetrics and Gynecology 1986; 67: 665–669

20. Ridsdale L. Evidence-based general practice: a critical reader. London: WB Saunders, 1995: 591–576

21. Giles JA, Hudson E, Crow J, Williams D, Walker P. Colposcopic assessment of the accuracy of cervical cytological screening. British Medical Journal 1988; 296; 1099–1102

22. Woodman CBJ, Yates M, Ward K, Williams D, Tomlinson K, Luesley D. Indicators of effective cytological sampling of the uterine cervix. Lancet 1989; ii: 88–90

23. Martin-Hirsch P, Lilford R, Jarvis G, Kitchener HC. Efficacy of cervical smear collection devices: a systematic review and meta-analysis. Lancet 1999; 354: 1763–1770

24. Wolfendale M. Cervical samplers: most important variable is probably the operator's skill. British Medical Journal 1991; 302: 1554–1555

25. Duguid HLD. Does mild atypia on a cervical smear warrant further investigation. Lancet 1986; ii: 1225

26. Buntix, F, Brouwers M. Relation between sampling device and detection of abnormality in cervical smears: a meta-analysis of randomised and quasi-randomised studies. British Medical Journal 1996; 313: 1285–1290

27. Klinkhamer P, Vooijs G, de Haan A. Intra-observer variability in the quality assessment of cervical smears. Acta Cytologica 1989; 33: 215–218

28. Vet de H, Knipschild P, Schouten H et al. Interobserver variation in histo-pathological grading of cervical dysplasia. Journal of Clinical Epidemiology 1990; 43: 1395–1398

29. Chomet J. Screening for cervical cancer: a new scope for general practitioners? Results of the first year of colposcopy in general practice. British Medical Journal 1987; 294: 1326–1328

30. IARC Working Group on evaluation of cervical cancer screening programmes. Screening for squamous cervical cancer: duration of low risk after negative results of cervical cytology and its implications for screening programmes. British Medical Journal 1986; 293: 656–664

31. Mitchell H, Medley G, Drake M. Quality control measures for cervical cytology laboratories. Acta Cytologica 1988; 32: 288–292

32. Van der Graaf Y, Voojis PG. False negative rates in cervical cytology. Journal of Clinical Pathology 1987; 40: 438–442

33. Sasieni PD, Cuzick J, Lynch-Farmery E, NCN Working Group. Estimating the efficacy of screening by auditing smear histories of women with and without cervical cancer. British Journal of Cancer 1996; 73: 1001–1005

34. Working Party of the Royal College of Pathologists. Achievable standards, benchmarks for reporting, criteria for evaluating cervical pathology. Cytopathology 1995; 6: 301–303

35. Buntinx F, Knottnerus J, Crebolder H, Seegers T, Essed G, Schouten H. Does feed-back improve the quality of cervical smears? A randomised controlled trial. British Journal of General Practice 1993; 43: 194–198

36. Laverty C, Farnsworth A, Thurloe J, Bowditch R. The reliability of a cytological prediction of cervical adenocarcinoma in situ. Australian and New Zealand Journal of Obstetrics and Gynaecology 1988; 28: 307–312

37. Williams EMI, Vessey MP. Compliance with breast cancer screening achieved by the Aylesbury Vale Mobile Service (1984–88). Journal of Public Health Medicine 1990; 12(1): 51–55

38. Pill R, French J, Harding K, Stoff N. Invitation to attend a health check in a general practice setting: comparison of attenders and non-attenders. Journal of the Royal College of General Practitioners 1988, 38: 53–56

39. Townsend P, Davidson N, Whitehead M. Inequalities in health. London: Penguin, 1988

40. Torgerson DJ, Donaldson C. An economic view of high compliance as a screening object. British Medical Journal 1994; 308: 117–119

41. Jenkins D, Gallivan S, Sherlaw-Johnson C, Patnick J, Austoker J. Compliance in screening programme: high compliance essential in cervical screening programme. British Medical Journal 1994; 308: 652–653

42. Jepson R, Clegg A, Forbes C, Lewis R, Sowden A, Kleijnen J. The determinants of screening uptake and interventions for increasing uptake: a systematic review. Health Technology Assessment Reports 2000; 4(14): iv–vii

43. Miller AB, G Anderson, J Brisson, et al. Report of a national workshop on screening for cancer for the cervix. Canadian Medical Association Journal 1991; 145(10): 1301–1325

44. Miller AB, Chamberlain J, Day NE, Hakama M, Prorock PC, eds. Cancer Screening International Union Against Cancer. Cambridge: Cambridge University Press 1991

45. Van Wijngaarden WJ, Duncan ID. Upper age limit for cervical screening. British Medical Journal 1993; 306: 1409–1410

46. Wilkinson C. Peters TJ, Harvey IM, Stott NCH. Risk targeting in cervical screening: a new look at an old problem. British Journal of General Practice 1992; 42: 435–438

47. Brinton LA. Epidemiology of cervical cancer – overview. In: Munoz N, Bosch FX, Shah KV, Meheus A, eds. The epidemiology of human papilloma virus and cervical cancer. International Agency for Research on Cancer, IARC Lyon Scientific Publication no. 119, 1992: 3–23

48. Murphy M, Mant D, Goldblatt P. Social class, marital status and cancer of the uterine cervix in England and Wales. 1950–83. Journal of Epidemiology and Community Health 1992; 46: 378–381

49. Knox EG. Ages and frequencies for cervical cancer screening. British Journal of Cancer 1976; 34: 444–452

50. Frame PS. Determinants of cancer screening frequency: the example of screening for cervical cancer. Journal of the American Board of Family Practice 1998; 11(2): 87–95

51. Parkin DM, Moss SM. An evaluation of screening policies for cervical cancer in England and Wales using a computer simulation model. Journal of Epidemiology and Community Health 1986; 40: 143–153

52. Oortmarsen GJ Van, Habbema J, Dik F, Ballegooijen M Van. Predicting mortality from cervical cancer after negative smear test results. British Medical Journal 1992; 305: 449–451

53. Herbert A, Stein K, Bryant TN et al. Relation between the incidence of invasive cervical cancer and the screening interval: is a five year interval too long? Journal of Medical Screening 1996; 3: 140–145

54. Waugh N, Robertson A. Costs and benefits of cervical screening II. Is it worth reducing the screening interval from five to three years? Cytopathology 1996; 7: 241–248

55. Bryant J, Stevens A. Cervical screening interval. R&D Directorate, South and West Regional Health Authority, 1995

56. Koopanschap MA, Lubbe KT, Van Ortmarssen GJ et al. Economic aspects of cervical screening. Social Science and Medicine 1990; 30: 1081–1087

57. Hakaman M, Miller AB, Day NE, eds. Screening for cancer of the uterine cervix. IARC Scientific Publication no. 76. Lyon: IARC, 1986: 133–142

58. Austoker J. Cervical screening in primary care: guidelines for working with primary care. Oxford: NHSCSP, 1990

59. Robertson JH, Woodend BE, Crozier EH, Hutchinson J. Risk of cervical cancer associated with mild dyskaryosis. British Medical Journal 1988; 297: 18–21

60. Campion MJ, Cuzick J, McCance DJ, Singer A. Progressive potential of mild cervical atypia: prospective cytological, colposcopic and virological study. Lancet 1986; ii: 237–40

61. Flannelly G, Anderson D, Kitchener HC, Mann EMF, Campbell M, Fisher F, Walker F, Templeton AA. Management of women with mild and moderate cervical dyskaryosis. British Medical Journal 1994; 308: 1399–1403

62. Shafi M. Controversies in management: management of women with mild dyskaryosis. Cytological surveillance avoids overtreatment. British Medical Journal 1994; 309: 590–592

63. Fox H. Cervical smears: new terminology and new demands. British Medical Journal 1987; 294: 1307–1308

64. Wilkinson C, Jones JM, McBride J. Anxiety caused by abnormal result of a cervical smear test: a controlled trial. British Medical Journal 1990; 300: 440

65. Baxter K, Peters T, Somerset M, Wilkinson C. Anxiety amongst women with mild dyskaryosis: costs of an educational intervention. Family Practice 1999; 16(4): 353–359

66. Wilkinson C, Jones JM, McBride J. Anxiety caused by abnormal result of a cervical smear test: a controlled trial. British Medical Journal 1990; 300: 440

67. Foster P, Anderson CM. Reaching targets in the national screening programme: are current practices unethical? Journal of Medical Ethics 1998; 24(3): 151–157

68. McCormick J. Medical ethics and the public health: the ethical dimension. Journal of Clinical Epidemiology 1996; 49: 619–621

69. Quinn MJ, Babb PJ, Jones J. Screening and mortality from cervical cancer. British Medical Journal 1999; 319: 642

70. National Audit Office. The performance of the NHS cervical screening programme in England: report by the comptroller and auditor general. London: Stationery Office, 1998

71. Finance and Performance Assessment Framework. Quality and performance in the NHS: high level performance indicators. Leeds: NHS Executive, 1999

72. Haward R, Goldacre M, Mason A, Willkinson E, Amess M, eds. Health outcome indicators: breast cancer. Report of a working group to the Department of Health. Oxford: National Centre for Health Outcomes Development, 1999

Family planning and contraception

Clare Seamark

Importance

In the UK the majority of women will be registered with a general practitioner (GP) for their medical and contraceptive care. There is free state provision of contraception through GP services (except condoms) and family planning clinics. Despite this, unintended and unwanted pregnancies still occur.[1–3] Many of these pregnancies will be terminated and the number of terminations of pregnancy in England and Wales reached its highest level of 187 401 in 1998.[4] Figures for 1997 would suggest that over 20% of pregnancies are terminated.[4,5] In comparison with women who have planned pregnancies, women who continue an unintended pregnancy may be more likely to suffer antenatal and postnatal depression, be less satisfied with their care and more likely to have postnatal health problems.[3] There has been great emphasis in recent years on teenage conceptions and targets have been set to reduce unwanted pregnancies in this age group.[6,7] However, there are numerically more terminations of pregnancy among women aged 20–24 years and the needs of older women also need to be considered. Rates of pregnancy, particularly among older teenagers, have not increased over the last 30 years although the age at first intercourse has decreased, so it is likely that there has been some impact from contraceptive services.[8] However, many women still do not use contraception early in their sexual experience or do not use effective methods regularly.[9–13]

Review of evidence relating to quality indicators

Screening for risk of unintended pregnancy

In the UK the majority of women receive contraceptive advice from their GP.[14–17] This places a responsibility on GPs to remain up to date with current contraceptive options and practice. Providing contraceptive advice is outside a GP's general medical services work and at the current time is reimbursed by a separate item of service claim. Some family planning services are provided opportunistically, during consultations for other matters. There is no evidence to support specific screening for unintended pregnancy although the risk of this should be considered at consultations with women of childbearing age. The availability and accessibility of a flexible and confidential service is important in providing a good-quality service.[18,19]

Treatment

Most effective methods of contraception can be obtained from general practice and from family planning clinics. The following reversible methods are available within UK general practice although all methods may not be available in every practice: combined oral contraceptive pills (COCs); progestogen only pills (POPs); intrauterine contraceptive devices and intrauterine system (Mirena: progestogen containing); injectable progestogens (Depo-Provera); progestogen implants (currently Implanon); diaphragms/caps and contraceptive jelly/spermicides. Condoms are not prescribable by GPs, but may sometimes be made available under local arrangements and can be obtained free from family planning clinics. Some GPs will offer a vasectomy service and there should be free access to both male and female sterilisation, and arrangements for referral for termination of pregnancy.

For the purposes of this review it has been decided to use prescription of COCs as the index for the quality indicators. This is because it is the most widely used method of reversible contraception, with currently about 26% of women of reproductive age (16–49 years) in the UK using it.[20] Nearly half of women using reversible contraception choose to use the COC. This means that about 3 million women will be using COCs each year, the majority of whom will obtain it from their GP.

The COC has been extensively studied since its introduction. Overall use of the COC would not appear to have an effect on mortality.[21–23] It produces some health benefits such as improved cycle control and decreased loss at menstruation. It also offers protection against endometrial and ovarian cancer.[21,23] However, it has also been associated with some health risks and these have become a focus for much attention. Much of the earlier work on the COC was on higher dose pills (ethinyl oestradiol or equivalent, of 50 μg or above) and some of the risks and benefits may differ with the newer lower dose pills (35 μg or below). The possible problems associated with the COC will be discussed with a view to the indicators that can be used to minimise the risks.

Venous thromboembolism (VTE)

Venous thromboembolism (VTE) was one of the first recognised risks of the COC that came from early case control studies[24,25] and which had initially been suspected by a GP in a letter to *The Lancet* in 1961, although he thought the thrombosis might have been due to dehydration and vomiting caused by the pill.[26] The early reports found a 4- to 9-fold increase in the risk of VTE in women using the COCs then available (50 μg ethinyl oestradiol: first-generation COCs). Since those studies, the dose of ethinyl oestradiol in COCs has been reduced to 35 μg or below, and this probably reflects the smaller (3- to 4-fold) relative risk in today's users.[27] There was concern, particularly in the UK in 1995 when it was suggested that COCs containing desogestrel and gestodene (so-called third-generation COCs) had a greater (possibly 2-fold) risk of VTE over the COCs containing levonorgestrel and norethisterone (so-called second-generation COCs).[28–30] This is still the subject of debate with some suggesting that the results are due to bias. It is now accepted that any difference must be small and the third-generation COCs have again been granted a first-line licence in the UK with the proviso that the possible small increase in VTE should be discussed.[31] Recent evidence from the UK has shown that there has been no significant change in the incidence of VTE despite a large decrease in the use of third-generation COCs.[32] It should also be remembered that the risk of VTE in pregnancy far exceeds that associated with any COC.

The risk factors for VTE in any woman include age, obesity, recent surgery and thrombophilias. Women starting the COC would need to have these taken into account. Screening for some of the commoner hereditary clotting defects such as factor V Leiden mutation has been suggested, but with low incidence of this disease and with 50% of cases of VTE occurring in women without a currently known clotting defect this is not a practical proposition.[33,34]

Most studies have not shown an association between VTE and current cigarette smoking, varicose veins or high blood pressure.[27] However, in others a small effect of smoking has been suggested.[29]

Although it is important to take a personal and family history for VTE risk from potential users of the COC this may not be recorded in such a way in the medical record as to be accessible for quality assessment.

Myocardial infarction

The risk of myocardial infarction (MI) in women of reproductive age is extremely small. Recently it has been shown that women who do not smoke and have no other risk factors are at little or no increased risk from taking the COC.[35,36] The differences that have been shown in past studies probably reflect the increased risk of women who smoke and those who have undetected high blood pressure with a possible 20-fold increase in risk for heavy smokers on the COC.[37] Recent studies have confirmed that smoking is an independent risk factor for MI and a probable additive effect when taking the COC[35] (indicator 1). Hypertension is another risk factor for MI and in some studies women who had not had blood pressure (BP) checked before starting the COC appeared to have a higher relative risk than women whose BP had been checked and were not hypertensive (indicator 3). Malignant hypertension on the COC has also been reported.[38] As MI is still a very rare event in young women, smoking is not usually seen as an absolute contraindication to taking the COC. By the time a woman is in her mid-30s her individual risk has risen and the added risk of smoking and the COC is usually judged to have reached the level at which if smoking is continued then ongoing use of the COC is not advised[35,39-41] (indicator 2). Others have found less influence from COCs with smoking being the major risk factor for MI in young women. However, patterns of smoking may have changed, use of lower dose COCs may also influence this and follow-up was not complete (60%).[42] Some might see light smoking (<15–20 cigarettes/day) as only a relative contraindication, but in this case clear records of discussion of this with the woman should be made, and most would veer on the side of caution, particularly if they feel that the amount of smoking may be underestimated (indicator 2). Some experts have suggested looking at other risk factors such as family history and lipid profiles before prescribing COCs for lighter smokers.[41]

Cerebrovascular disease

Cerebrovascular disease is also extremely rare in women of reproductive age. There is a small increased risk in low-risk women (non-smoking, non-hypertensive women who have had their BP checked before prescription for the COC) of ischaemic stroke of about 1.5 times that of non-users.[39,43] Hypertension is again an independent risk factor, increasing the risk at least 3 times over COC users without hypertension (indicators 3 and 4). Smoking again is a risk factor in women who do not use the COC and increases the risk 2- to 3-fold for women who take the COC[39,43] (indicators 1 and 2). There are no obvious differences among the different low-dose COC preparations.[44]

Migraine has been shown to be another independent risk factor for ischaemic stroke. It is thought that this risk is further increased in a woman who takes the COC.[45] A recent statement on the use of COCs in women with migraine has suggested the following absolute contraindications to COC use: migraine with aura (focal neurological symptoms precede headache; if this is present before a request for COC it should not be used, or if it occurs when on the COC the pill should be stopped immediately) (indicator 5); migraine without aura but with more than one additional risk factor for stroke; severe migraine/'status migrainosus' attacks lasting more than 72 hours before or after using the COC; and migraine treated with ergot derivatives. Women with migraine without aura should also be counselled for other risk factors.[46]

There does not appear to be any increased risk of haemorrhagic stroke in non-smokers under the age of 35 years without hypertension who take the COC. Again hypertension and smoking are independent risk factors for stroke, increasing the risk for women using the COC by 10 times for hypertension and 3 times for smoking[39] (indicators 1, 2, 3 and 4).

Carcinoma of the breast

It is possible that there may be a slight increased risk of carcinoma of the breast in women who use the COC. This may be related to young age at starting and taking the COC for many years. At present this risk has not been adequately quantified and the rate of breast cancer in older women has not increased in line with the possible effect that might be expected.[47]

Carcinoma of the cervix

It has been suggested that use of the COC increases the risk of cervical cancer,[48] and a small increase in relative risk has been associated with duration of use.[23] In many cases this has been hard to distinguish from the other known risk factors for cervical cancer such as young age at commencement of sexual intercourse, multiple partners or smoking. At present there are no extra recommendations apart from encouraging all women in the target age group for cervical screening (currently 20–65 years in the UK) to have regular smears taken.[49] There is no indication for routine screening of teenagers even when they are sexually active.[50]

Recommended quality indicators for family planning and contraception

Treatment
1 Women prescribed COCs should be asked about their current smoking status
2 Women over the age of 35 who smoke should not be prescribed COCs without justification
3 A woman's blood pressure should be measured when she starts the COC or have been recorded within the previous 12 months
4 Women prescribed the COC should have their blood pressure checked within 6 months of starting COC
5 Women with a history of migraine with aura should not be prescribed the COC

Overview of data sources used in this review

This review is based on information from the following sources: the WHO publication, *Improving Access to Quality Care in Family Planning*; evidence-based books published on family planning and sexual health care in primary care in the UK; research papers published in the 1990s relating to the risks and benefits of the combined oral contraceptive pill (COC). The COC is used as the index method of contraception for this review, since it is the most commonly used method in general practice.

Further reading

Carter Y, Moss C, Weyman A, eds. *RCGP handbook of sexual health in primary care.* London: RCGP, 1998

Drife JO. *Benefits and risks of oral contraception today,* 2nd edn. Pantheon, 1996

Guillebaud J. *Pill and other forms of hormonal contraception.* Oxford Paperbacks, 1999

Guillebaud J. *Contraception your questions answered,* 3rd edn. London: Churchill Livingstone, 1999

Rowlands S. *Managing family planning in general practice.* Oxford: Radcliffe Medical Press, 1997

Szarewski A, Guillebaud J. *Contraception – a user's handbook,* 2nd edn. Oxford University Press, Oxford, 1998

World Health Organization. *Improving access to quality care in family planning. Medical eligibility for contraceptive use.* Geneva: WHO, 1996

References

1. Allaby MAK. Risks of unintended pregnancy in England and Wales in 1989. British Journal of Family Planning 1995; 21: 93–94
2. Fleissig A. Unintended pregnancy and the use of contraception: changes from 1984–1989. British Medical Journal 1991; 302: 147
3. Fleissig A. A rise in 'unintended' babies. What are the implications? British Journal of Family Planning 1994; 19: 260–263
4. Office for National Statistics. Abortion Statistics. Series AB no. 25. London: ONS, 1998
5. Office for National Statistics. Birth statistics. Series FM1 no. 26. London: ONS, 1997
6. Secretary of State. The health of the nation. A strategy for health in England. London: HMSO, 1992
7. Social Exclusion Unit. Teenage pregnancy. London: Stationery Office, 1999

8. Wellings K, Kane R. Trends in teenage pregnancy in England and Wales: how can we explain them? Journal of the Royal Society of Medicine 1999; 99: 277–282

9. Pollack AE. Teen contraception in the 1990s. Journal of School Health 1992; 62: 288–293

10. Wellings K, Field J, Johnson A, Wadsworth J. Sexual behaviour in Britain. Harmondsworth: Penguin, 1994

11. Griffiths M. Contraceptive practices and contraceptive failures among women requesting termination of pregnancy. British Journal of Family Planning 1990; 16: 16–18

12. Houghton A. Knowledge of contraception in abortion seekers compared with other pregnant and non-pregnant women. British Journal of Family Planning 1994; 20: 69–72

13. Pearson VAH, Owen MR, Phillips DR, Gray DJP, Marshall MN. Pregnant teenagers' knowledge and use of emergency contraception. British Medical Journal 1995; 310: 1644

14. Department of Health. Health and personal social services statistics for England. London: HMSO, 1993

15. Johnson C, Madeley JR. Contraceptive care in a general practice. British Journal of Family Planning 1995; 21: 52–54

16. Seamark CJ, Gray DJP. Do teenagers consult general practitioners for contraceptive care? British Journal of Family Planning 1995; 21: 50–51

17. Rowlands S. Contraceptive use in a rural general practice. Journal of the Royal Society of Medicine 1998; 91: 297–300

18. Rowlands S. Managing family planning in general practice. Oxford: Radcliffe Medical Press, 1997

19. Carter Y, Moss C, Weyman A, eds. RCGP handbook of sexual health in primary care. London: RCGP, 1998

20. Office for National Statistics. Contraception and sexual health. London: ONS, 1997

21. Hannaford PC, Kay CR. The risk of serious illness among oral contraceptive users: evidence from the RCGP's contraceptive study. British Journal of General Practice 1998; 48: 1657–1662

22. Skegg DCG. Editorial. Oral contraception and health. British Medical Journal 1999; 318: 69–70

23. Beral V, Hermon C, Kay C, Hannaford P, Darby S, Reeves G. Mortality associated with oral contraceptive use: 25 year follow up of 46,000 women from the Royal College of General Practitioner's oral contraception study. British Medical Journal 1999, 310: 96–100

24. Royal College of General Practitioners. Oral contraception and thromboembolic disease. Journal of the Royal College of General Practitioners 1967; 13: 267–279

25. RCGP Oral Contraceptive Study. Combined pill, venous thrombosis and varicose veins. Journal of the Royal College of General Practitioners 1978; 28: 393–399

26. Jordan WM. Pulmonary embolism (letter). Lancet 1961; ii: 1146–1147

27. WHO Collaborative study of cardiovascular disease and steroid hormone contraception. Venous thromboembolic disease and combined pill: results of an international multicentre case control study. Lancet 1995; 346: 1575–1582

28. WHO Collaborative study of cardiovascular disease and steroid hormone contraception. Effect of different progestogens in low oestrogen containing oral contraceptives on venous thromboembolism. Lancet 1995; 346: 1582–1588

29. Jick H, Jick SS, Gurewich V, Myers MW, Vasilakis C. Risk of idiopathic cardiovascular death and nonfatal venous thromboembolism in women using oral contraceptives with differing progestagen components. Lancet 1995; 346: 1589–1593

30. Spitzer WO, Lewis MA, Heinemann LAJ, Thorogood M, MacRae KD on behalf of Transnational Research Group on Oral Contraceptives and the Health of Young Women. Third generation oral contraceptives and risk of venous thromboembolic disorders: an international case-control study. British Medical Journal 1999; 312: 83–88

31. Committee on Safety of Medicines and Medicines Control Agency. Combined oral contraceptives containing desogestrel or gestodene and the risk of venous thromboembolism. Current Problems in Pharmacovigilance 1999; 25: 12

32. Farmer RDT, Williams TJ, Simpson EL, Nightingale AL. Effect of 1995 pill scare on rates of venous thromboembolism among women taking combined oral contraceptives: analysis of General Practice Research Database. British Medical Journal 2000; 321: 477–479

33. Bloemenkamp KWM, Rosendaal FR, Helmerhorst FM. Enhancement by factor V Leiden mutation of risk of deep venous thrombosis associated with oral contraceptives containing a third generation progestogen. Lancet 1995; 346: 1593–1596

34. Machin SJ, Mackie IJ, Guillebaud J. Factor V Leiden mutation, venous thromboembolism and combined oral contraceptive usage. British Journal of Family Planning 1995; 21: 13–14

35. WHO Collaborative study of Cardiovascular Disease and Steroid Hormone Contraception. Acute myocardial infarction and combined oral contraceptives: results of an international multicentre case-control study. Lancet 1997; 349: 1202–1209

36. Dunn N, Thorogood M, Faragher B et al. Oral contraceptives and myocardial infarction: results of the MICA case-control study. British Medical Journal 1999; 318: 1759–1784

37. Croft P, Hannaford PC. Risk factors for acute myocardial infarction in women: evidence from Royal College of General Practitioners' oral contraception study. British Medical Journal 1989; 298: 165–168

38. Lim KG, Isles CG, Hodsman GP, Lever AF, Robertson JWK. Malignant hypertension in women of childbearing age and its relation to the contraceptive pill. British Medical Journal 1987; 294: 1057–1058

39. WHO collaborative study of cardiovascular disease and steroid hormone contraception. Haemorrhagic stroke – overall stroke risk and combined oral contraceptives: results from an international multicentre case-control study. Lancet 1996; 348: 505–510

40. Mishell DR Jr. Cardiovascular risks: perception versus reality. Contraception 1999; 59 (suppl): 21S–24S

41. Schiff I, Bell WR, Davis V et al. Oral contraceptives and smoking, current considerations: recommendations of a consensus panel. American Journal of Obstetrics and Gynecology 1999; 180(6 pt 2): S383–S384

42. Dunn NR, Faragher B, Thorogood M et al. Risk of myocardial infarction in young female smokers. Heart 1999; 82: 581–583

43. Heinemann LAJ, Lewis MA, Thorogood M, Spitzer WO, Guggenmoos-Holzmann I, Bruppacher R and the Transnational Research Group on Oral Contraceptives and the Health of Young Women. Oral contraceptives and the risk of thromboembolic stroke. British Medical Journal 1997; 315: 1502–1504

44. Crook D. Do different brands of oral contraceptives differ in their effects on cardiovascular disease? British Journal of Obstetrics and Gynaecology 1997; 104: 516–520

45. Chang CL, Donaghy M, Poulter N. Migraine and stroke in young women: case-control study. The World Health Organisation Study of Cardiovascular Disease and Steroid Hormone Contraception. British Medical Journal 1999; 318: 13–18

46. MacGregor EA, Guillebaud J. Recommendations for clinical practice – combined oral contraceptives, migraine and ischaemic stroke. British Journal of Family Planning 1998; 24: 53–60

47. Collaborative Group on Hormonal Factors in Breast Cancer. Breast cancer and hormonal contraceptives: collaborative reanalysis of individual data on 53,297 women with breast cancer and 100,239 women without breast cancer from 54 epidemiological studies. Lancet 1996; 347: 1713–1727

48. Fitzgerald C, Elstein M. Editorial. The oral contraceptive and cervical neoplasia. British Journal of Family Planning 1995; 20: 79–80

49. Hannaford PC, Webb AMC. Evidence-guided prescribing of combined oral contraceptives: consensus statement. Contraception 1996; 54: 125–129

50. Olamijulo J, Duncan ID. Is cervical cytology screening of teenagers worthwhile? British Journal of Obstetrics and Gynaecology 1995; 102: 515–516

▶20

Hormone replacement therapy

Jean Coope

Importance

The menopause is the permanent cessation of menstruation resulting from loss of ovarian follicular activity.[1] The diagnosis is usually based on an accurate history but it may need to be confirmed biochemically in young women with amenorrhoea, in women after hysterectomy who have had their ovaries conserved, and in women taking oral contraceptives or hormone replacement therapy before menopause (where cyclical bleeding is artificially induced). FSH levels >30 u/L indicate menopause but fluctuating levels can occur in the perimenopausal period. Some authorities recommend that FSH levels should be measured annually after a simple hysterectomy.[2]

The average age of menopause worldwide is 51 years[3] and the average life expectancy after menopause is now 30 years. Endogenous oestrogen declines at menopause and there is an associated increase in osteoporosis, bone fracture and cardiovascular disease. Vasomotor symptoms occur in 50–85% of women at the time of menopause. These symptoms are influenced by cultural factors, for example Japanese women have a low incidence of symptoms.[4] In addition to the vasomotor symptoms, about 45% of women over the age of 60 have symptoms of urogenital atrophy.

Review of evidence relating to indicators

Screening

Screening for menopause in patients where the diagnosis is doubtful is appropriate for women at high risk of complications of the menopause but other groups can be assessed on the basis of age and symptoms.

Treatment

Hormone replacement therapy for relief of menopausal symptoms

Hormone replacement therapy (HRT) is effective for the relief of vasomotor symptoms, insomnia[5] and urogenital atrophy associated with menopause[6,7,7a] (indicator 3). Local oestrogen is effective for urethral and vaginal problems such as vaginal dryness and atrophy. Progestogens and tibolone are effective in controlling flushes.

Sexual drive is unaffected by natural menopause[8] but early castration can result in severe loss of libido due to loss of ovarian androgens. This is treatable using testosterone.[9] Continuing sexual activity helps to protect against vaginal atrophy. Dyspareunia, vaginal irritation and pain can be treated with local oestrogen cream or use of a vaginal ring.[10] One controlled study suggested that vaginal oestriol reduced the incidence of urinary tract infections[11] but this finding was not confirmed subsequently.[12] Progestogen supplements are unnecessary with low-dose local oestrogen but postmenopausal bleeding should always be investigated.

Depression

It is unclear whether menopause causes depression or whether HRT is an effective treatment for depressive symptoms.[13–15] It does appear, however, that disturbed sleep is significantly related to mood changes at the time of menopause.[16] Although there is some evidence that early menopause (before the age of 40 years) is associated with depressive illness,[17] the consensus is that there is insufficient evidence to link normal menopause with clinical depression.[18]

Prevention

Osteoporosis

Osteoporosis is a major cause of pain, disability and death. There are 200 000 osteoporotic fractures each year in the UK at a cost of £942 million. 1 in 3 women and 1 in 12 men over the age of 50 years will have an osteoporotic fracture.[19] HRT prevents the rapid phase of bone loss after the menopause and maintains bone mass for the duration of treatment in most women[20] (indicator 4). Women at increased risk of osteoporosis and fractures are those with:

▶ early fragility fracture

▶ oophorectomy or natural menopause under the age of 45 years

▶ prolonged amenorrhoea before menopause[21]

▶ prednisolone or equivalent at a dose greater than 7.5 mg for 3 months or more[22]

▶ thyroid disease[23]

▶ malabsorption[23a]

▶ rheumatoid arthritis.[22]

The risk of fracture is related directly to bone density. If bone mineral density (BMD) indicates a high fracture risk and HRT is inappropriate or unacceptable, bisphosphonates or raloxifene can be used. Quantitative ultrasound offers safe, low-cost assessment in general practice. It is a strong predictor of fracture risk but is best used in conjunction with DEXA.[23]

Observational studies show a 25% reduction in relative risk (RR) of fracture in women who have ever used HRT.[24,25] There is a small proportion of women in whom it has no effect on osteoporotic changes[26] but the majority of studies have shown significant benefits for the prevention of osteoporosis.[27–29] Current users starting HRT at menopause have an RR of 0.29 for hip fracture but the effect diminishes rapidly 5 years after stopping treatment.[30] Michaëlsson et al[31] concluded that recent use offers the greatest protection. In current users, therapy started 9 years after menopause was found to be as effective as treatment started at the time of menopause. Since the median age of fracture is 79 years,[24] long-term HRT extending into old age is likely to be the most effective form of prevention of osteoporosis risk.

Coronary heart disease

Heart disease caused over 78 000 deaths among British women in 1991. The incidence rises after the menopause 2-fold compared with premenopausal women of the same age.[32] Observational studies report a lower risk of coronary heart disease (CHD) in postmenopausal oestrogen users compared with non-users[24,33] and HRT is now recommended by most observers for primary prevention of CHD.[34–36] The principal mechanism of action is via the lipid profile, by increasing HDL cholesterol, lowering LDL cholesterol and reducing levels of total cholesterol.[37] However, there is still some debate about the risk:benefit ratio[38] and about the role of the progesterone component of combined preparations. Trials are currently being conducted to examine the relative benefits of oestrogens alone and combined preparations on the risk of CHD. Observational evidence suggests no association between stroke and the use of HRT.[39]

While the evidence linking HRT to reduced risk of CHD is strong, the potential selection bias of observational studies should be recognised, since women at lower risk are more likely to use HRT and to be non-smokers.[40–42]

The only published randomised controlled trial of HRT in women with pre-existing coronary disease (secondary prevention) does not support treatment with HRT. 2763 women with coronary disease younger than 80 years randomly received HRT or placebo.[43] Follow-up for 4.1 years showed a significant increase in CHD events in the first year, though there were fewer incidents in HRT users in years 4 and 5. Over the whole period of the study there was no difference between the treatment and control groups. HRT is therefore not recommended for secondary prevention of CHD, though women already on treatment should probably be advised to continue.

There is no evidence that HRT affects blood pressure. Nevertheless, taking the blood pressure of women before and during treatment is generally regarded as good practice (indicators 1 and 2).

Cancer of the colon

There is some evidence that HRT users are at lower risk of colon cancer than non-users.[44]

Alzheimer's disease

Observational studies suggest that Alzheimer's dementia may be less common in HRT users than among controls,[45–48] but other studies have suggested that HRT does not protect against dementia[49] and oestrogen is not recommended for prevention or treatment of Alzheimer's disease or other dementias until adequate trials have been completed.

Risks of hormone replacement therapy

Endometrial cancer

Women with an intact uterus experience an increased risk of irregular bleeding, endometrial hyperplasia and endometrial cancer if they use unopposed oestrogens[50] (indicator 5). A meta-analysis of 30 observational studies demonstrated an overall relative risk of endometrial cancer of 2.3 for oestrogen users compared with non-users, rising to 9.5 after 10 years of use.[51] Mortality from endometrial cancer also increased among oestrogen users.

Continuous or cyclical (for 12 days each month) progestogen used in conjunction with the oestrogens eliminates the increased risk.[6,52] Taking progestogen for only 10 days each cycle reduces but does not eliminate the increased risk.[53] Oestradiol implants necessitate the use of long-term progestogen.[54]

Women should receive a pelvic examination before starting HRT to ensure that there is no uterine enlargement or other abnormal pelvic masses.[1,55] Routine endometrial sampling before starting HRT is unnecessary, however.

Ovarian cancer

There is no evidence of an increased risk of ovarian cancer in HRT users.[3]

Vulval cancer

There is no evidence of an increased risk of vulval cancer in HRT users.[3]

Breast cancer

International data based on 52 705 breast cancer patients and 108 411 controls concluded that the risk of breast cancer increases with duration of use of HRT.[56] This excess risk reduces when therapy is withdrawn and disappears 5 years after stopping HRT. Between the ages of 50 and 70 years the cumulative incidence of breast cancer is 45 per 1000 in never-users of HRT. This risk is increased by 2 cases per 1000 women after 5 years of use, by 6 cases per 1000 after 10 years of use and by 12 cases per 1000 after 15 years of use. Swedish studies have confirmed an RR of between 1.4 and 2.43 after 10 years of HRT use.[57,58] Progestins do not reduce the risk and there is some evidence that they may actually increase it.[59]

Obesity and weight gain are confounding factors in observational studies linking HRT to increased risk of breast cancer, since both are strongly associated with postmenopausal breast cancer. In a cohort of 95 000 nurses followed up for 16 years, the RR was 1.99 for women with a weight gain of greater than 20 kg in comparison with women with unchanged weight.[60]

Women with a first-degree relative with premenopausal breast cancer also have an increased risk of developing the disease and the question arises as to the safety of HRT for these women. However, 8 years follow-up of over 41 000 women in Iowa showed that in those with a family history of breast cancer, HRT was not associated with an added increased incidence compared with never-users.[61] Benign breast disease does not contraindicate HRT.[62]

Many women who recover from stage 1 breast cancer then suffer menopausal symptoms. Until recently breast cancer was regarded as a contraindication for HRT but various studies have failed to show an increased mortality in women with a personal history of breast cancer who have taken HRT. An 8-year survey of 2600 breast cancer survivors found the probability of dying to be 0.14 among non-users and past users and 0.09 among current users.[63] HRT users who develop breast cancer are more likely than non-users to have a favourable histology,[64] the tumours are more likely to be small[65–67] and the survival rate higher than in non-users.[68] As early menopause before the age of 40 lowers the risk of breast cancer,[69] HRT should be prescribed long-term in this group. Since there are ethical and medicolegal dilemmas when prescribing HRT for women with a history of breast cancer, treatment should be based on informed consent of the patient and agreed with specialists[70,71] (indicator 6).

Most authorities and manufacturers guidelines emphasise the importance of breast awareness and regular mammograms for women on HRT[72,73] (indicator 2). However, HRT reduces the sensitivity and specificity of screening mammography.[74–78] Indirect evidence supports clinical examination carried out after training,[79] though the Department of Health has advised against routine breast examination and suggested that it should not be delegated to a nurse.

In summary, the consensus on good practice is that initial assessment should include enquiry about personal and family history of breast cancer or symptoms, e.g. lump or bleeding, and breast examination by a doctor.[1] Mammography and/or specialist referral is indicated if there are positive history or findings, or extreme anxiety. Routine pretreatment mammography is not recommended in the UK but patients should attend for 3-yearly NHS mammography screen. Self-examination is of unproven benefit but breast awareness can be taught by a nurse.[30a]

Thromboembolism

Early studies demonstrated accelerated blood clotting in women on conjugated equine oestrogen[80,81] and an increased risk of thromboembolism in women currently taking HRT was found in 1996[82–85]. A relative risk of venous thromboembolism in women on HRT of between 2.1 and 3.6 has been reported in case controlled studies.[38,82–86] The Committee on Safety of Medicines[87] advised that the baseline risk of thromboembolism for non-users of HRT is 1 per 10 000 per year which increased to 3 per 10 000 for current users of HRT.

Particular caution is needed when treating women with a personal or family history of deep vein thrombosis, obesity, trauma or prolonged bedrest. In these high-risk groups laboratory screening for thrombophilia may be helpful[88] but a negative screen should not give false reassurance in women with a personal history of venous thrombotic disease, since they are at considerable risk of recurrence.[1]

Recommended quality indicators for hormone replacement therapy

---

Screening and diagnosis

1 Prior to patients starting HRT treatment a doctor or nurse should undertake:
   a. history (including counselling about the risks and benefits)
   b. blood pressure check
2 Patients on HRT should be:
   a. offered a review including history (including side-effects, counselling about duration of treatment) and examination (BP) at least annually
   b. encouraged to take part in a national mammography screening programme

Treatment

3 Patients suffering from vasomotor symptoms at or after menopause should be offered HRT if other causes are excluded and there are no contraindications
4 Women with early menopause (<45 years), FH osteoporosis, long-term use or repeated courses (>3 times a year) of prednisolone >7.5 mg/day, early fragility fracture (vertebral fracture without any trauma, fracture neck of femur without major trauma [simple fall is not major trauma]), malabsorption, or rheumatoid arthritis should be offered HRT unless there are specific contraindications
5 Women with an intact uterus should not be offered unopposed oestrogen unless the patient has tried and is unable to tolerate oestrogen plus progestogen or tibolone, or unless endometrial sampling is performed periodically
6 Patients with a history of breast cancer should not be offered HRT except following referral for specialist opinion
7 Women with a history of deep vein thrombosis or pulmonary embolism should not be offered HRT unless the risks and benefits have been discussed

---

Overview of data sources used in this review

This review is based on evidence from the 1996 US Preventative Services Task Force (USPSTF) and 1992 ACOG technical bulletin on HRT, Medline review articles 1990–7 and under MeSH headings, Hormone Replacement Therapy and relevant secondary subjects, the Cochrane Library, and a search of the following journals from 1997 to April 2000: *New England Journal of Medicine*; *Journal of the American Medical Association*; *British Medical Journal*; *Lancet*; and *British Journal of Obstetrics and Gynaecology*.

Further reading

Rees M, Purdie DW, eds. Management of the menopause. BMS Publications, 1999

Department of Health. Advisory group on osteoporosis. G89/003 4051 1AR 5k. London: DOH, 1994

Department of Health. Quick reference primary care guide on the prevention and treatment of osteoporosis. 3362 HSD 30k 1P. London: DOH, 1998

Effective Health Care. Screening for Osteoporosis to prevent Fractures. University of Leeds, 1992

National Osteoporosis Society. Information for health care professionals. PO BOX 10, Barton Meade House, Radstock, Bath BA3 3YB, NOS, 1998

National Osteoporosis Society. Accidents, falls, fractures and osteoporosis. PO BOX 10, Barton Meade House, Radstock, Bath BA3 3YB, 1999

National Osteoporosis Society. The primary care group (PCG) service framework on osteoporosis. NOS: Osteoporosis Review 2000; 8(1)

Prescribers' Journal. The Stationery Office 2000; 40(2)

Royal College of Physicians. Osteoporosis: Clinical guidelines for the prevention and treatment. London: RCP, 1999

Rymer J, Morris EP. Clinical evidence. BMJ Publications, 1999

University of Leeds. Effective health care (1992) (1) B

United States Preventative Task Force. Guide to clinical preventive services. 2nd edn. Baltimore MD. Williams & Wilkins, 1996

World Health Organization. Research on the menopause in the 1990s. Geneva: WHO, 1996

References

1. Rees M, Purdie DW, eds. Management of the menopause. BMS Publications, 1999
2. Seeley T. Oestrogen treatment therapy after hysterectomy. British Medical Journal 1992; 305: 811–812
3. World Health Organization. Research on the monopause in the 1990s. Geneva: WHO, 1996: 71–72
4. Lock M. Contested meanings of the menopause. Lancet 1991; 337: 1270–1272
5. Antoni Jevic IA, Stalla GK, Steiger A. Modulation of sleep electroencephalogram by estrogen replacement in postmenopausal women. American Journal of Obstetrics and Gynecology 2000; 182: 277–282
6. Belohotz PF. Hormonal treatment of postmenopausal women. New England Journal of Medicine 1994; 330(15): 1062–1071
7. Coope J Hormonal and non-hormonal interventions for menopausal symptoms. Maturitas 1996; 23: 159–168
7a. PEPI. Writing Group for the PEPI Trial. Journal of the American Medical Association 1995; 273; 199–208
8. Leiblum S, Bachmann G, Kemmann E et al. Vaginal atrophy in the postmenopausal woman. Journal of the American Medical Association 1983; 249(16): 2195–2198
9. Burger H, Hailes J, Nolson J, Menelaus M. Effect of combined implants of oestradiol and testosterone on libido in postmenopausal women. British Medical Journal 1987; 294; 936–937
10. Lose G, Engler E (2000). Oestradiol-releasing vaginal ring v. oestriol vaginal pessaries in treatment of bothersome lower urinary tract symptoms. British Journal of Obstetrics and Gynaecology 2000; 107: 1029–1034
11. Raz R, Stamm WE. A controlled trial of intravaginal estriol in postmenopausal women with recurrent urinary tract infections. New England Journal of Medicine 1993; 329: 753–756
12. Cardozo L, Benness C, Abbott D. Low dose oestrogen prophylaxis for recurrent urinary tract infections in elderly women. British Journal of Obstetrics and Gynaecology 1998; 105(4): 403–407
13. McKinlay SM, Brambilla DJ, Posner JG. The normal menopause transition. Maturitas 1992; 14: 103–115
14. Kaufert PA, Gilbert P, Tate R. The Manitoba Project: a re-examination of the link between menopause and depression. Maturitas 1992; 14: 143–155
15. Hunter MS. Emotional well-being, sexual behaviour and hormone replacement therapy. Maturitas 1990; 12: 299–314
16. Baker A, Simpson S, Dawson D. Sleep disruption and mood changes associated with menopause. Journal of Psychosomatic Research 1997; 43(4): 359–369
17. Harlow BL, Cramer DW, Annis JM. Association of medically treated depression and age at natural menopause. American Journal of Epidemiology 1995; 141(12): 1170–1176
18. Nicol-Smith L Causality, menopause and depression: critical view of the literature. British Medical Journal 1996; 313(7067): 1229–1232
19. National Osteoporosis Society. Accidents, falls, fractures and osteoporosis. 1999
20. Department of Health. Report: Advisory group on osteoporosis. London: DOH, 1994
21. Davies MC, Hall ML, Jacobs HS Bone mineral loss in young women with amenorrhoea. British Medical Journal 1990; 301: 790–793

22. Spector TD, Hall GM, McCloskey EV, Kanis JA. Risk of vertebral fracture in women with rheumatoid arthritis. British Medical Journal 1993; 306: 558

23. Franklyn JA, Sheppard MC. Thyroxine replacement treatment and osteoporosis. British Medical Journal 1990; 300: 693–694

23a. National Osteoporosis Society. Information for health care professionals: The use of quantitative ultrasound in the management of osteoporosis in primary or secondary care. 1998

24. Grady D, Rubin S, Petitti DB et al. Hormone therapy to prevent disease and prolong life in postmenopausal women. Annals of Internal Medicine 1992; 117(12): 1016–1037

25. Maxim P, Ettinger B, Spitalny GM Fracture protection provided by long-term estrogen treatment. Osteoporosis- Int. 1995; 5(1): 23–29

26. World Health Organization. Assessment of fracture risk and its application to screening for postmenopausal osteoporosis. WHO Study Group report. Geneva: WHO 1994

27. PEPI. Effects of hormone therapy on bone mineral density. Journal of the American Medical Association 1996; 276(17): 1389–1396

28. Schneider DL, Barrett-Connor EL, Morton DJ. Timing of post-menopausal estrogen for optimal bone mineral density. Rancho Bernado Study. Journal of the American Medical Association 1997; 277(7): 543–547

29. Felson DT, Zhang Y, Hannan MT et al. The effect of postmenopausal estrogen therapy on bone density in elderly women. New England Journal of Medicine 1993; 329: 1141–1146

30. Cauley JA, Seeley DG, Ensrud K et al. Estrogen replacement therapy and fractures in older women. Study of Osteoporotic Fractures Research Group. Annals of Internal Medicine 1995; 122(I): 9–16

30a. Department of Health. Examination of the breasts. Ph/CNO/98/1. London: DOH, 1998

31. Michaëlsson K, Baron JA, Farahmand BY et al. Hormone replacement therapy and risk of hip fracture: population based case-control study. British Medical Journal 1998; 316: 1858–1863

32. Kannell WB,Hjortland MC, McNamara PM, Gordon T. Menopause and risk of cardiovascular disease: the Framingham Study. Int Med 1976; 85: 447–452

33. Stampfer J, Colditz GA, Willett WC et al. Postmenopausal estrogen therapy and cardiovascular disease. New England Journal of Medicine 1991; 325: 756–762

34. Grodstein F, Stampfer MJ, Manson JE et al. Postmenopausal estrogen and progestin use and the risk of cardiovascular disease. New England Journal of Medicine 1996; 335(7): 453–461

35. Grodstein F, Stampfer MJ, Colditz GA et al. Postmenopausal hormone therapy and mortality. New England Journal of Medicine 1997; 336(25): 769–775

36. Sourander L, Rajala T, Raiha I et al. Cardiovascular and cancer morbidity and mortality and sudden cardiac death in postmenopausal women on oestrogen replacement therapy (ERT). Lancet 1998; 352: 1965–1969

37. Espeland MA, Marcovina SM, Miller V et al. Effect of postmenopausal hormone therapy on lipoprotein(a) concentration. (PEPI). Circulation 1998; 97(10): 979–986

38. Hemminki E, McPherson K. Value of drug-licensing documents in studying the effects of postmenopausal hormone therapy on cardiovascular disease. Lancet 2000; 355: 566–569

39. Grodstein F, Stampfer MJ, Goldhaber SZ et al. Prospective study of exogenous hormones and risk of pulmonary embolism in women. Lancet 1996; 348(9003): 983–987

40. Coope J, Roberts D. A clinic for the prevention of osteoporosis in general practice. British Journal of General Practice 1990; 40: 295–299

41. Hemminki E, Malin M, Topo P. Selection to postmenopausal therapy by women's characteristics. Journal of Clinical Epidemiology 1993; 46(3): 211–219

42. Rödström K, Bengtsson C, Lissner L, Björkelund C. Pre-existing risk-factor profiles in users and non-users of hormone replacement therapy; prospective cohort study in Gothenburg, Sweden. British Medical Journal 1999; 319: 890–893

43. Hulley S, Grady D, Bush T et al. Randomized trial of estrogen plus progestin for secondary prevention of coronary heart disease in postmenopausal women. Journal of the American Medical Association 1998; 280(7): 605–613

44. Prihartono N, Palmer JR, Louik C et al. A case-control study of use of postmenopausal female hormone supplements in relation to the risk of large bowel cancer. Cancer Epid Biom Prev 2000; 9 (4): 443–447

45. Paginini-Hill A. Oestrogen replacement therapy and Alzheimer's disease. British Journal of Obstetrics and Gynaecology 1996; 103(13): 80–86

46. Tang M-X, Jacobs D, Stern Yaakov et al Effect of oestrogen on risk and age at onset of Alzheimer's disease. Lancet 1996; 348: 429–432

47. Kawas C, Resnick S, Morrison A et al. A prospective study of estrogen replacement therapy and the risk of developing Alzheimer's disease; the Baltimore Study of Aging. Neurology 1997; 48(6): 1517–1521

48. Baldereschi M, Di-Carlo A, Lepore V et al. Estrogen-replacement therapy and Alzheimer's disease in the Italian Longitudinal Study on Aging. Neurology 1998; 50(4): 996–1002

49. Barrett-Connor E, Kritz-Silverstein D. Estrogen replacement therapy and cognitive function in older women. Journal of the American Medical Association 1993; 269(20): 2637–2641

50. Lethaby, A Farquhar C, Sarkis A, Roberts H, Jepson R, Barlow D. The association of oestrogen, oestrogen-progestogen and placebo with endometrial hyperplasia and irregular bleeding in the menopause. The Cochrane Library, Issue 3, 1999

51. Grady D, Gebretsadik T, Kerlikowske K et al. Hormone replacement therapy and endometrial cancer risk: a meta-analysis. Obstetrics and Gynecology 1995; 85(2): 304–313

52. PEPI. Effects of hormone replacement therapy on endometrial histology in postmenopausal women. The Writing Group for the PEPI Trial. Journal of the American Medical Association 1996; 275(5): 370–375

53. Beresford SAA, Weiss NS, Voigt LF, McKnight B. (1997) Risk of endometrial cancer in relation to use of oestrogen combined with cyclic progestogen therapy in postmenopausal women. Lancet 1997; 349: 458–461

54. Gangar KF, Fraser D, Whitehead MI, Cust MP. Prolonged endometrial stimulation associated with oestradiol implants. British Medical Journal 1990; 300: 436 438

55. Spencer CP, Whitehead MI. British Journal of Obstetrics & Gynaecology. Review: endometrial assessment re-visited. 1999; 106: 623–632

56. Collaborative Group on Hormonal Factors in Breast Cancer. Breast cancer and hormone replacement therapy: collaborative reanalysis of data from 51 epidemiological studies of 52,705 women with breast cancer and 108,411 women without breast cancer. Lancet 1997; 350: 1047–1059

57. Persson I, Thurfjell E, Bergstrom R, Holmberg L. Hormone replacement therapy and the risk of breast cancer. Nested case control study in a cohort of Swedish women attending mammography screening. International Journal of Cancer 1997; 72(5): 758–761

58. Magnusson C, Baron JA, Correia N, Bergstrom R, Adami HO. Breast cancer risk following long-term oestrogen and oestrogen-progestin replacement therapy. International Journal of Cancer 1999; 81(3): 339–344

59. Schairer C, Roisi H, Lubin J et al. Menopausal oestrogen and estrogen-progestin replacement therapy and breast cancer risk. Journal of the American Medical Association 2000; 283 (4) 485–491

60. Huang Z, Hankinson SE, Graham A et al. Dual effects of weight and weight gain on breast cancer risk. Journal of the American Medical Association 1997; 278: 1407–1411

61. Collore TA, Mink PJ, Cerhan JR et al. The role of hormone replacement therapy in the risk for breast cancer and total mortality in women with a family history of breast cancer. Annals of Internal Medicine 1997; 127: 973–980

62. Dupont WD, Page DL, Parl FF et al. Estrogen replacement therapy in women with a history of proliferative breast disease. Cancer 1999; 85(6): 1277–1283

63. Schairer C, Gail M, Byrne C et al. Estrogen replacement therapy and breast cancer survival in a large screening study. Journal of the National Cancer Institute 1999; 91(3): 264–270

64. Gapstur SM, Morrow M, Sellers TA. Hormone replacement therapy and risk of breast cancer with a favorable histology. Journal of the American Medical Association 1999; 281: 2091–2097

65. Magnusson C, Holmberg L, Norden T et al Prognostic characteristics in breast cancers after hormone replacement therapy. Breast Cancer Research and Treatment 1996; 38(3): 325–334

66. Holli K Isola J, Cuzick J. Low biologic aggressiveness in breast cancer in women using hormone replacement therapy. Journal of Clinical Oncology 1998; 16(9): 3115–3120

67. Salmon RJ, Ansquer Y, Asselain B et al. Clinical and biological characteristics of breast cancer in post-menopausal women receiving hormone replacement therapy for menopause. Oncol Rep. 1999; 6(3): 699–703

68. Jernstrom H, Frenander J, Ferno M, Olsson H. Hormone replacement therapy before breast cancer diagnosis significantly reduces the overall death rate compared with never-use among 984 breast cancer patients. British Journal of Cancer 1999; 80(9): 1453–1458

69. Titus-Ernstoff L, Longnecker MP, Newcomb PA et al. Menstrual factors in relation to breast cancer risk. Can Epid. Biomark Prev 1998; 7(9): 783–789

70. Birkhauser M. Hormone replacement therapy and estrogen-dependent cancers. Int J Fertil Meo Stud 1994; 39(2): 99–114

71. Anon. British Journal of General Practice. Editorial: The use of HRT in patients with breast cancer: yes, no, or sometimes. 2000; 50: 454

72. Achuthan R, Parkin G, Horgan K. Screening mammography for women starting hormone-replacement therapy. Lancet 1999; 353: 1855

73. British National Formulary. British Medical Association. Royal Pharmaceutical Society of Great Britain (2000)

74. Laya MB, Larson EB,Taplin SH, White E. Effect of estrogen replacement therapy on the specificity and sensitivity of screening mammography. Journal of the National Cancer Institute 1996; 88(10): 643–649

75. Kavanagh AM, Mitchell H, Giles GG. Hormone replacement therapy and accuracy of mammographic screening. Lancet 2000; 355: 270–274
76. Litherland JC. Stallard S, Hole D, Cordiner C. The effect of hormone replacement therapy on the sensitivity of screening mammograms. Clinical Radiology 1999; 54(5): 285–288
77. Greendale GA, Reboussin BA, Sie A et al. Effects of estrogen and estrogen-progestin on mammographic parenchymal density (PEPI). Annals of Internal Medicine 1999; 130(4 pt 1): 262–269
78. Beral V Banks E, Reeves G et al. Correspondence: hormone replacement therapy and high incidence of breast cancer between mammographic screens. Lancet 1997; 349: 1103–1104
79. Barton MB, Harris R, Fletcher SW. Does this patient have breast cancer. Journal of the American Medical Association 1999; 282: 1270–1280
80. Coope J, Thomson JM, Poller L. Effects of 'natural oestrogen' replacement therapy on menopausal symptoms and blood clotting. British Medical Journal 1975; 4: 139–143
81. Poller L, Thomson JM, Coope J. Conjugated equine oestrogen and blood clotting: a follow-up report. British Medical Journal 1977; 1: 935–936
82. Daly E, Vessey MP, Hawkins MM et al Risk of venous thromboembolism in users of hormone replacement therapy. Lancet 1996; 348: 977–980
83. Jick H, Derby LE, Myers MW et al. Risk of hospital admission for idiopathic venous thromboembolism among users of postmenopausal oestrogen. Lancet 1996; 348: 981–983
84. Gutthann SP, Rodriguez LAG, Castellsague J, Oliart AD Hormone replacement therapy and risk of venous thromboembolism: population based case-control study. British Medical Journal 1997; 514: 796–800
85. Varas LC, Rodriguez LAG, Cattaruzzi C et al. Hormone replacement and the risk of hospitalization for venous thromboembolism: a population based study in southern Europe. American Journal of Epidemiology 1998; 147(4): 387–390
86. Oger E, Scarabin PY. An assessment of the risk for venous thromboembolism among users of hormone replacement therapy. Drugs and Aging 1999; 14(l): 55–61
87. Committee on Safety of Medicines. Current problems in pharmaco-vigilance: a risk of venous thromboembolism with hormone replacement therapy. Medicines Control Agency 1996; 22: 9–10
88. Scottish Medicines Resource Centre. Hormone replacement therapy: new products. 1996; 33: 127–129

▶21

Immunisations

Alison Round

Importance

In deriving quality indicators for immunisation, a number of considerations are relevant. These are:

▶ the importance of the disease that immunisation is intended to prevent

▶ the evidence that immunisation against a particular disease is both efficacious in a trial situation and effective in usual practice

▶ the evidence that primary care practice can influence the uptake of immunisation

▶ the feasibility of using various measures for monitoring immunisation programmes, ideally from routine or easily available sources.

The uptake of childhood immunisations in the UK is generally high and the written record of childhood immunisation may be held outside a child's general practitioner records. This review therefore focuses on the evidence for three vaccine-preventable diseases of the greatest public health importance in the UK generally given to adults: hepatitis B, influenza and pneumococcal disease.

How immunisations work

Immunisations are the primary method of preventing many communicable diseases in the UK. They work both by inducing immunity in the recipient (individual immunity) and by creating herd immunity in a community that has a high level of vaccination. If more than a threshold percentage of a community is immunised, then the disease is unable to spread as there are insufficient numbers of susceptible individuals to maintain transmission.

Influenza, pneumococcal and hepatitis B are vaccines targeted at high-risk groups in the UK and protection with these vaccinations is individual.

Hepatitis B virus

Incidence and prevalence
The prevalence of hepatitis B is in the order of 1 in 2500 in new blood donors in the UK. The number of overt cases is low, at around 600 per year. Two-thirds of hepatitis B infections are asymptomatic and may not be diagnosed.

Natural history

About 2–10% of those infected as adults become chronic carriers with surface antigen persisting for longer than 6 months.[1] Around 20–25% of hepatitis B carriers develop progressive liver disease, leading in some patients to cirrhosis. The prognosis of the liver disease is not clear, although there is increased risk of developing hepatocellular carcinoma.

Transmission

Hepatitis B is transmitted parenterally and sexually. Transmission most commonly occurs following vaginal or anal intercourse, or as a result of sharing needles or other equipment among intravenous drug users. Perinatal transmission from mother to child also occurs.

High-risk groups

Most infections occur among those with behavioural or occupational risk factors. These are parenteral drug users, individuals who change sexual partners frequently, particularly homosexual and bisexual men, and men and women who are prostitutes. Close family contacts of the case, or carrier, are at risk, as are people with severe learning difficulties.

There is some evidence that needle exchange schemes are ineffective in reducing hepatitis B prevalence among drug users.[2,3]

Influenza

Incidence and prevalence

Around 4000 deaths per year are attributed to influenza. In epidemic years, 20–50% of the population may be affected and there are a large number of excess deaths, mainly among elderly people. Epidemics occur unpredictably, as influenza viruses change antigens and populations have little immunity to the new subtypes.

Natural history

Influenza affects all age groups and is usually a self-limiting disease with recovery in 2–7 days. It is characterised by mild respiratory symptoms but severe systemic symptoms can occur. It may be complicated by bronchitis, bacterial pneumonia and otitis media.

Transmission

Influenza is highly infectious with an incubation period of 1–3 days. An affected individual sheds large numbers of virus and hence influenza spreads rapidly.

High-risk groups

Elderly people with chronic respiratory and cardiac disease are most susceptible.

Invasive pneumococcal disease

Incidence and prevalence

Pneumococcal disease is a major cause of morbidity and mortality, accounting for 2000–14 000 deaths in the UK each year.

Natural history
The pneumoccocus is the commonest cause of community-acquired pneumonia, but can also result in bacteraemia, septicaemia, otitis media and meningitis.

Transmission
The bacterium is transmitted by respiratory aerosol. The incubation period is short, typically 1–5 days.

High risk groups
Pneumococcal disease is particularly severe among the very young, the elderly or those with impaired immunity or an absent or non-functioning spleen.

Adverse effects

Despite the success of vaccination programmes, public awareness of and controversy about vaccine safety has increased. Media coverage of potential adverse effects of vaccination has a marked effect on immunisation uptake. There is scientific consensus that for all currently recommended vaccination programmes, vaccination is safer than accepting the risks for the diseases that the vaccines prevent.[4,5]

Review of evidence relating to indicator set

The effectiveness of a vaccination programme depends on interrupting the transmission between an affected and a susceptible individual. Selective vaccination programmes rely not only on the effectiveness of the specific vaccination for an individual, but also on the uptake of vaccination among those groups deemed to be at risk.

Hepatitis B vaccination
Hepatitis B vaccination has been available since 1981 but has had little impact on the incidence of disease.[2] Estimated efficacy of the current recombinant vaccine is between 80% and 90%.[6] Trials in high-risk groups show protection of about 67% (95% CI 21–93%).[7] However, uptake is poor among homosexual men and drug users.[8,9]

One retrospective study[3] and one cohort study[10] evaluated the effectiveness of hepatitis B vaccination in drug users. Vaccination was associated with an 89% reduction in viral antigen seroprevalence in the former and a 66% serological response to vaccination in the latter. It is likely that these changes will translate into longer term health benefits. However, this is partly dependent on the length of effectiveness of vaccination.

Influenza vaccine
Influenza vaccine is prepared each year using virus strains considered most likely to be circulating the forthcoming winter. Annual immunisation is necessary with vaccine containing the most recent strains.

A recent meta-analysis identified 20 cohort trials, 3 case control studies and 1 randomised controlled trial estimating the effect of influenza vaccine on elderly persons.[11]. These showed approximately 50% efficacy in preventing respiratory illness, pneumonia and hospitalisation, and a 68% reduction in mortality. A subsequent randomised controlled trial[12] showed similar results in people infected with human immunodeficiency virus (HIV).

Pneumococcal vaccine

The current pneumococcal vaccine is a polysaccharide capsule derived preparation. This formulation of vaccine is much less effective than conjugate vaccines, such as that used against haemophilia influenza type B.

A meta-analysis of randomised controlled trials was published in 1994[13] and included 9 trials and 40431 patients. This review suggested a 66% reduction in definite pneumococcal pneumonia, but only a small reduction in all-cause pneumonia. There was no reduction in mortality. There was no apparent effect in high-risk patients.

A more recent meta-analysis concluded that there was an overall reduction in invasive pneumococcal disease of 73% following vaccination, which was effective in high-risk patients.[14] However, subsequent trials not included in this meta-analysis have been less positive.[15–18]

None of these studies showed any protection for people with impaired humoral immunity.[18,19] People with anatomic asplenia do appear to receive about 85% protection, based on an extremely small number of cases.[20] However, British Clinical Haematology guidelines recommend pneumococcal vaccination for patients with splenectomy regardless of immune status.[21]

There is uncertainty about the effectiveness of pneumococcal vaccination. Although there seems to be some benefit in healthy and immunocompetent adults, these are not the groups of people who are generally offered vaccination. The degree of protection for patients at a higher risk is uncertain. A new conjugate vaccine is being developed which appears to be more effective.[22]

Current policy

As these vaccinations are given to high-risk adults, there is a necessity to maintain a register of eligible individuals for each separate vaccination and to have a suitable recall system in order to achieve high coverage rates. Influenza vaccination has a different formulation each year and cannot be produced rapidly in large amounts. In the case of hepatitis B, the at-risk group may not be easily defined as behavioural characteristics are not routinely recorded in most medical records. Several reports document low uptake rates in these high-risk groups.[23]

There is no fee for service for these adult immunisations in primary care. The only financial incentive is by purchasing immunisations at a lower cost than reimbursement. If more immunisations are purchased than used, there can be a financial loss for general practices.

Box 21.1 shows the Joint Committee on Vaccination and Immunisation recommended groups for receipt of hepatitis B, influenza and pneumococcal vaccinations (indicators 1, 2, 3 and 4).

Box 21.1   High-risk groups in whom vaccination is recommended

Hepatitis B
Babies born to mothers who are chronic carriers of hepatitis B or who have had acute hepatitis
    B during pregnancy*
Parenteral drug misusers
People who change sexual partners frequently
Close family contacts of a case or carrier
Families adopting children from countries with a high prevalence of hepatitis B
Haemophiliacs or those receiving regular blood products
Patients with chronic renal failure
Health care staff who come into contact with blood or body fluids
Staff working at and residents of institutions caring for the severely learning disabled
Inmates and staff of custodial institutions
Those travelling to areas of high prevalence for lengthy periods

Influenza
Chronic respiratory disease
Chronic heart disease
Chronic renal failure
Diabetes
Immunosuppression of any cause
Residents of institutions
Anyone aged over 65**

Pneumococcal
Asplenia or severe splenic dysfunction
Chronic respiratory disease
Chronic heart disease
Chronic renal failure or nephrotic syndrome
Immunosuppression of any cause
Chronic liver disease
Diabetes

---

* Screening of pregnant women recommended in HSC 1998/127
** Recommended in communication from Department of Health, May 2000

Evidence of interventions to increase uptake in primary care

Interventions to increase uptake in primary care can be categorised into three groups. The first is community- or society-based interventions such as mass media campaigns or legal systems requiring proof of vaccination before entry to school. These interventions will not be covered here as they are not considered to be under the control of primary care. The second category is individual patient-based interventions, which may or may not be administered through primary care. The third category is primary care organisational-based interventions of a number of different types. The latter two categories form the basis of this section. Most research has been carried out in the USA, which may be of limited relevance in the UK. Only randomised comparisons are included.

Individual-based interventions

These consist of patient reminder or recall systems, either alone or supplemented by other interventions. A reminder is an unsolicited communication with the patient suggesting that vaccination is now due or is recommended. In some cases a reminder alone was used; in others the reminder was part of a larger strategy to increase vaccination rates.

Evidence for patient reminders alone

Influenza vaccination
Fourteen randomised studies of patient reminders, ranging from a personal letter signed by the physician to a mailed brochure, demonstrated a decrease in uptake (1 study only) of 7% in the intervention group, to increases of between 1% and 31%. The median increase was 6%.[24–38]

Pneumococcal vaccine
One randomised trial has shown an increase of 13% in vaccine uptake.[39]

Hepatitis B vaccination
One randomised trial in a high-risk group (attenders at a sexually transmitted disease clinic who had already agreed to vaccination) showed a 23% increase in completed vaccination rates for a telephone reminder in addition to mailed reminders.[40] The effect was most marked in people with low educational attainment.

Effectiveness of patient reminders used in combination with other interventions
Comparison with the patient reminders alone trials suggests a greater effect for multicomponent strategies.

Influenza vaccination
There are 10 randomised studies looking at influenza vaccination in this category. One showed a decrease in uptake of 8%, but the others showed increases ranging from 2% to 47%[28,41–49]. The median increase in uptake was 16%.

Pneumococcal vaccine
One study considered effects on pneumococcal vaccination. The effect was a 21% increase in uptake.[49]

Hepatitis B vaccination
There are no trials relating to the uptake of hepatitis B vaccination.

Interventions based in primary care

Increasing patient information

Influenza vaccination
Three randomised studies considered influenza and the provision of education or information, showing a range from a decrease in uptake of 2%, to an increase of 17%.[50-52]

Pneumococcal vaccine
Three studies included pneumococcal vaccine, and showed increases in uptake of 2%, 16% and 16%.[50,51,53]

Hepatitis B vaccination
One study provided information to students about hepatitis B vaccination and reported an increase in uptake of 9%.[54]

Patient-held records
The evidence for patient-held medical records as an intervention is equivocal. For influenza there was no difference in one trial[55] and an 18% increase in uptake in another, which showed no effect on pneumococcal vaccine rates.[56]

Interventions to improve the convenience of, or access to vaccination

Four studies showed effects ranging from no effect[57] to 37% increase in uptake for influenza and 82% increase in uptake for pneumococcal vaccine.[45,58,59]

Physician reminders
An effect was demonstrated in one study for hepatitis B but not for influenza or pneumococcal immunisation.[60]

Summary of evidence to improve uptake of vaccinations

There is good evidence that reminder or recall systems improve the uptake of vaccinations by a moderate amount. Providing information alone to patients does not seem to have an effect, but improving access to vaccinations may have a modest effect. Multicomponent interventions appear to have greater effect than single interventions.

Recommended quality indicators for immunisations

Hepatitis B

1 Adults and adolescents in the high-risk groups should be offered 3 doses of hepatitis B vaccine within 1 year of the following risk factors:
   a. babies of mothers who are chronic carriers of hepatitis B
   b. babies who have had acute hepatitis B during pregnancy
   c. parenteral drug misusers
   d. haemophiliacs or those receiving regular blood products
   e. patients with chronic renal failure on dialysis

Influenza

2 Adults and adolescents in the following high-risk groups should be offered an annual influenza vaccination:
   a. chronic respiratory disease
   b. chronic heart disease
   c. chronic renal failure
   d. diabetes
   e. immunosuppression of any cause
   f. residents of nursing and residential homes
   g. anyone aged over 75

Pneumococcal

3 Adults and adolescents in the high-risk groups except splenectomy should receive pneumococcal vaccination on one occasion:
   a. asplenia or severe splenic dysfunction
   b. chronic respiratory disease
   c. chronic heart disease
   d. chronic renal failure or nephrotic syndrome
   e. immunosuppression of any cause
   f. chronic liver disease
   g. diabetes
4 Adults and adolescents who have no spleen should have received pneumococcal vaccine within the last 10 years

---

Overview of data sources used in this review

In the UK the Joint Committee of Vaccinations and Immunisations (JCVI) produces recommendations for immunisation schedules for national programmes and immunisations intended for high risk groups. Recommendations are published every 4–5 years in the 'Green Book' *Immunisation against Infectious Disease.*[6] Changes to policy are published in *CDR Weekly* and disseminated to all GPs via health authority cascade mechanisms.

In addition, Medline, Embase and the Cochrane Library were searched for systematic reviews and controlled clinical trials considering the effectiveness of hepatitis B, influenza and pneumococcal vaccination policies and the effects of interventions to improve or maintain vaccine coverage. The primary care influence on uptake of vaccination draws heavily on the US Task Force on Community Preventive Services review[61] and a search made for work subsequent to this. Studies were included if they were randomised controlled trials and provided information on comparative immunisation rates in two groups. A literature review, 'Quality of health care for children and adolescents',[62] produced by the RAND Corporation was also used as a source document.

References

1. Edmunds WJ, Medley GF, Nokes DJ, Hall AJ, Whittle HC. The influence of age on the development of the hepatitis B carrier state. Proceedings of the Royal Society of London Biological Sciences 1993;253:197–201
2. Balogun MA, Ramsay MA, Firlay CK, Collins M, Hepunstall J. Acute hepatitis B infection in England and Wales: 1985–96. Epidemiology and Infection 1999; 122(1): 659–666
3. Lamden KH, Kennedy M, Beeching NJ et al. Hepatitis B and hepatitis C virus infections: risk factors among drug users in north west England. Journal of Infection 1998; 37(3): 260–269
4. Anon. MMR vaccine coverage shows signs of recovery. Communicable Disease Reports Weekly 1999: 9; 345
5. Anon. Update: vaccine side effects, adverse reactions, contraindications, and precautions. Recommendations of the Advisory Committee on Immunization practices. Morbidity and Mortality Weekly Report 1996; 6(45 RR-12): 1–35
6. Salisbury DM, Begg NT. Immunisation against infectious disease, 2nd edn. London: HMSO, 1996
7. Jefferson T et al. Vaccines for preventing hepatitis B in health care workers. Cochrane Review, 1997
8. Anderson B, Bodsworth NJ, Rorsheim R.A. Hepatitis B virus infection and vaccination status of high risk people in Sydney: 1982 and 1991. Medical Journal of Australia 1995; 161(6): 368–371
9. McKusker J, Hill EM, Mayer, KH. Awareness and use of hepatitis B vaccine among homosexual male clients of a Boston community health centre. Public Health Reports 1990; 105(1): 59–64
10. Minniti F, Baldo V, Trivello R, Bricolo R, Di Furia L, Renzulli G, Chiaramonte M. Response to HBV vaccine in relation to anti-HCV and anti-Hbc positivity: a study in intravenous drug addicts. Vaccine 1999; 17(23–24): 3083–3085
11. Gross PA, Hermogenes AW, Sacks HS, Lee J, Levandowski RA. The efficacy of influenza vaccine in elderly persons: a meta-analysis and review of the literature. Annals of Internal Medicine 1995; 123(7): 518–527
12. Tasker S, Treaner JJ, Paxton WB, Wallace MR. Efficacy of influenza vaccination in HIV infected persons. A randomized, double-blind, placebo-controlled trial. Annals of Internal Medicine 1999; 131(6): 430–433
13. Fine MJ, Smith MA, Carson CA et al. Efficacy of pneumococcal vaccination in adults: a meta-analysis of randomised controlled trials. Archives of Internal Medicine 1994; 154: 2666–2677
14. Hutchison BG, Oxman AD, Shannon HS, Lloyd S, Altmayer CA, Thomas K. Clinical effectiveness of pneumococcal vaccine. Meta-analysis. Canadian Journal of Family Practice 1999; 45: 2381–2393
15. Koivula I, Slen M, Leinones M, Makela PH. Clinical efficacy of pneumococcal vaccine in the elderly: A randomized, single-blind population-based trial. American Journal of Medicine 1997; 103(4): 281–290
16. Ortqvist A, Hedlund J, Burman LA et al. A randomised trial of 23 valent pneumococcal capsular polysaccharide vaccine in prevention of pneumonia in middle aged and elderly men. Lancet 1998; 351: 399–403
17. Hokanen PO, Keisttinene T, Miettinene L. Incremental effectiveness of pneumococcal vaccine on simultaneously administered influenza vaccine in preventing pneumonia and pneumococcal pneumonia among persons aged 65 or older. Vaccine 1999; 17: 2493–2500
18. French N, Nakigingi J, Coupenter LM et al. 23-valent pneumococcal polysaccharide vaccine in HIV-1-infected Ugandan adults: double-blind, randomised and placebo controlled trial. Lancet 2000; 355: 2106–2111
19. Nguyen-van-Tam JS, Neal KR. Clinical effectiveness, policies and practices for influenza and pneumococcal vaccines. Seminars in Respiratory Infection 1999; 14(2): 184–195
20. Bolan MD, Broome CV, Facklam RR, Plikyatis BD, Fraser DW, Schlech FW. Pneumococcal vaccine efficacy in selected poulations in the United States. Annals of Internal Medicine 1986; 104(1): 1–6
21. Working Party of the British Committee for Standards in Haematology Clinical Haematology Task Force. Guidelines for the prevention and treatment of infection in patients with an absent or dysfunctional spleen. British Medical Journal 1996; 312: 430–434

22. Black S, Shinefield H, Fireman B et al. Efficacy, safety, and immunogenicity of heptavalent pneumococcal conjugate vaccine in children. Pediatric Infectious Diseases Journal 2000; 19(3): 187–195

23. Edmunds WJ. Universal or selective immunisation against hepatitis B virus in the United Kingdom. Communicable Disease and Public Health 1998; 1(4): 221–228

24. Peuch M, Ward J, Lajoie V. Postcard reminders from GPs for influenza vaccine: are they more effective than an ad hoc approach? Australian and New Zealand Journal of Public Health 1998; 22(2): 254–256

25. Barnes G, McKinney W. Postcard reminders and influenza vaccination (letter). Journal of the American Geriatrics Society 1989; 37: 195

26. Buchner D, Larson E, White R. Influenza vaccination in community elderly: a controlled trial of postcard reminders. Journal of the American Geriatrics Society 1987; 35: 755–760

27. Clayton E, Hickson G, Miller C. Parents' responses to vaccine information pamphlets. Pediatrics 1994; 93: 369–372

28. Moran W, Wofford J, Velez R. Assessment of influenza immunization of community elderly: illustrating the need for community-level health information. Carolina Health Services Review 1995; 3: 21–29

29. Baker A, McCarthy B, Gurley V, Yood M. Influenza immunization in a managed care organization. Journal of General Internal Medicine 1998; 13(7): 469–475

30. Smith D, Zhou X-H, Weinberger M, Smith FM, Donald R. Mailed reminders for area-wide influenza immunization: a randomized controlled trial. Journal of the American Geriatrics Society 1999; 47(1): 1–5

31. Mullooly J. Increasing influenza vaccination among high-risk elderly: a randomized controlled trial of a mail cue in an HMO setting. American Journal of Public Health 1987; 77: 626–627

32. Brimberry R. Vaccination of high-risk patients for influenza: a comparison of telephone and mail reminder methods. Journal of Family Practice 1988; 26: 397–400

33. Anon. Increasing influenza vaccination rates for Medicare beneficiaries – Montana and Wyoming. Morbidity and Mortality Weekly Report 1994; 44: 741–744

34. Carter W, Beach L, Inui T. The flu shot study: using multi-attribute theory to design a vaccination intervention. Organizational behavior and Human Decision Processes 1986; 38: 378–391

35. Grabenstein J, Hartzema A, Guess HEA. Community pharmacists as immunisation advocates: a pharmacoepidemiologic experiment. International Journal of Pharmacy Practice 1993; 2: 5–10

36. Larson EB, Begama J, Hiedrich F, Alvin BL, Schneeweiss R. Do postcard reminders improve influenza compliance? A prospective trial of different postcard cues. Medical Care 1982; 20: 639–648

37. McDowell I, Newell C, Rosser W. Comparison of three methods of recalling patients for influenza vaccination. Canadian Medical Association Journal 1986; 135: 991–997

38. McDowell I, Newell C, Rosser W. A follow-up study of patients advised to obtain influenza immunizations. Family Medicine 1990; 22: 303–306

39. Siebers M, Hunt V. Increasing the pneumococcal vaccination rate of elderly patients in a general internal medicine clinic. Journal of the American Geriatrics Society 1985; 33: 175–178

40. Sellors J, Pickard L, Mahony J, Jackson K, Nelligan P, Zimic-Vincetic M, Chernesky M. Understanding and enhancing compliance with the second dose of hepatitis B vaccine: a cohort analysis and a randomized controlled trial. Canadian Medical Association Journal 1997; 157(2): 143–148

41. Moran W, Nelson K, Wofford JEA. Computer-generated mailed reminders for influenza immunization: a clinical trial. Journal of General Internal Medicine 1992; 7: 535–537

42. Becker D, Gomez E, Kaiser DEA. Improving preventive care at a medical clinic: how can the patient help? American Journal of Preventive Medicine 1989; 5: 353–359

43. Diaz Gravalos G, Palmeiro Fernandez G, Vazquez Fernandez L, Casado Gorriz I, Fernandez Bernardez M. Personalised appointments as a recruitment method for anti-flu vaccination in the elderly. Atencion Primaria 1999; 24(4): 220–223

44. Satterthwaite P. A randomised intervention study to examine the effect on immunisation coverage of making influenza vaccine available at no cost. New Zealand Medical Journal 1997; 110: 58–60

45. Karuza J, Calkins E, Feather JEA. Enhancing physician adoption of practice guidelines: dissemination of influenza vaccination guideline using a small-group consensus process. Archives of Internal Medicine 1995; 155: 625–632

46. Spaulding S, Kugler J. Influenza immunization: the impact of notifying patients of high-risk status. Journal of Family Practice 1991; 33: 495–498

47. Nexoe J, Kragstrup J, Ronne T. Impact of postal invitations and user fee on influenza vaccination rates among the elderly: a randomized controlled trial in general practice. Scandinavian Journal of Primary Health Care 1997; 15: 109–112

48. Buffington J, Bell K, LaForce F. A target-based model for increasing influenza immunizations in private practice. Genesee Hospital Medical Staff. Journal of General Internal Medicine 1991; 6: 204–209

49. Krieger JW, Castorina JS, Walls ML et al. Increasing influenza and pneumococcal immunization rates: a randomised controlled study of a senior center-based intervention. American Journal of Preventive Medicine 2000; 18(2): 123–131

50. Beck A, Scott J, Williams P, Robertston B, Jackson D, Gade G, Cowan P. A randomized trial of group outpatient visits for chronically ill older HMO members: the Cooperative Health Care Clinic. Journal of the American Geriatrics Society 1997; 45(5): 543–549

51. Herman C, Speroff T, Cebul R. Improving compliance with immunization in the older adult: results of a randomized cohort study. Journal of the American Geriatrics Society 1994; 42: 1154–1159

52. Kerse N, Flicker L, Jolley D, Arroll B, Young D. Improving the health behaviours of elderly people: Randomised controlled trial of a general practice. British Medical Journal 1999; 319(7211): 683–687

53. Jacobson TA, Thomas DM, Morton FJ et al. Use of a low literacy patient education tool to enhance pneumococcal vaccination rates. A randomised controlled trial. Journal of the American Medical Association 1999; 282(7): 646–650

54. Marron R, Lanphear B, Kouides R, Dudman L, Manchester R, Christy C. Efficacy of informational letters on hepatitis B immunization rates in university students. Journal of American College Health 1998; 47(3): 123–127

55. Dietrich A, Duhamel M. Improving geriatric preventive care through a patient hold checklist. Family Medicine 1089; 21: 195–198

56. Turner R, Waivers L, O'Brien K. The effect of patient-carried reminder cards on the performance of health maintenance measures. Archives of Internal Medicine 1990; 150: 645–647

57. Black M, Ploeg J, Walter SEA. The impact of a public health nurse intervention on influenza vaccine acceptance. American Journal of Public Health 1993; 83: 1751–1753

58. Dalby DM, Sellors JW, Fraser FD, Fraser C, van Ineveld C, Howard M. Effect of preventive home visits by a nurse on the outcomes of frail elderly people in the community: a randomized controlled trial. Canadian Medical Journal 2000; 162(4): 497–500

59. Rhew DC, Glasman PA, Goetz MB. Improving pneumococcal vaccine rates Nurse protocol versus clinical reminders. Journal of General Internal Medicine 1999; 14(6): 351–356

60. Flanagan JR, Doebbeling BN, Dawson J, Beekmann S. Randomized study of online vaccine reminders in adult primary care. Proceedings of AMIA Symposium, 1999: 755–759

61. Shefer A, Briss P, Rodewald L, Bernier R, Strikas Rea. Improving immunization coverage rates: an evidence-based review of the literature. Epidemiological Reviews 1999; 21(1): 96–142

62. McGlynn EA, Ansberg C, Kerr EA, Schuster M. Quality of care for children and adolescents: a review of selected clinical conditions and quality indicators. RAND Health Programme, 1997

▶ 22

How to use the quality indicator set

Martin Roland

Key points

▶ The quality indicators described in this book are aimed primarily at clinicians working in general practice, and at clinical governance leaders and managers working to improve the quality of care in primary care groups, trusts, health boards and local health groups ('primary care organisations')

▶ The prime purpose of quality indicators is to stimulate discussion about quality, not to make definitive judgements about it.

▶ We outline both the benefits and the risks of using quality indicators in general practice.

▶ We believe that quality indicators can have an important role in improving the quality of care provided in general practice. They can be also used to satisfy requirements for revalidation and clinical governance.

The indicators, with their associated literature reviews presented in Chapters 3–21, have been developed in order to be useful to those thinking about the assessment of quality in general practice. This includes general practitioners and practice nurses working within practices and the clinical and non-clinical managers working in primary care groups and trusts who have a wider responsibility for promoting quality improvement in primary care.

As outlined in Chapter 1, using indicators to assess quality of care has merits, but also has distinct drawbacks. In this final chapter we describe some of the ways in which these indicators might be used, along with some of the ways that they should not. As with any form of quality assessment, there are risks if the indicators are used without thought about what the results may or may not mean.

Operationalising the indicators

For indicators to be useful, they have to be expressed in a way that allows the clinical information to be collected easily. We hope that most of the indicators in this set are already clear and unambiguous. Some of them, however, are open to interpretation. For example, few would argue that for patients with diabetes, the diagnosis should be clearly marked in the medical records, so that any health professional who sees such a patient takes this into account (diabetes, indicator 1). But what does 'clearly marked' mean? How can this be operationalised to ensure that data are collected in a reliable way? We have produced a series of operational manuals to help standardise data collection and these are available on our website at www.npcrdc.man.ac.uk.

The scope of the indicator set

We believe that readers are likely to find the literature reviews at least as valuable as the proposed quality indicators. For many of the chosen conditions, we have not been able to produce quality indicators that cover more than a small part of the care of the condition. This may have been because there was insufficient evidence or lack of professional consensus, or because the expert panel members did not rate potential indicators sufficiently highly for them to be included in the final set. Back pain and acne are good examples. For conditions like these, doctors and nurses will be able to use the literature reviews to think about their own care, or to develop guidelines for use in their own practices. It is very important for those interpreting the indicators from outside practices to understand that they are not able to describe all important aspects of clinical care for any of the conditions – most clinicians will recognise this and it is important that non-clinicians do so as well.

It is also important to recognise that assessing clinical quality using indicators like those in this book only addresses one aspect of quality of care in general practice. This in turn represents only one aspect of quality in the broader arena of primary care. In the handbook *Quality Assessment in General Practice*[1] we have described how looking at clinical quality relates to other aspects of quality assessment and improvement. The handbook *Clinical Governance: A Guide for Primary Care Teams*[2] provides a list of internet based resources to support other quality issues, including evidence-based practice. In addition, a handbook that is aimed specifically at improving mental health care[3] is available, as is one for pharmacists working with practices to improve the quality of prescribing.[4] The text of these handbooks can be downloaded from the website of the National Primary Care Research and Development Centre at www.npcrdc.man.ac.uk.

Using the indicators in practices

We expect that the indicators in this book will most often be used by doctors and nurses in individual practices. Increasingly, clinicians want to think about their own performance. There are a number of reasons for this, but the one that is likely to dominate is the need to provide information to satisfy the requirements of clinical governance and evidence for revalidation of general practitioners. So, whereas the motivation for audit or other forms of quality assessment was largely internal, there is now an increasing expectation that general practitioners will use quality indicators to demonstrate to themselves and to others that they are providing good care.

Choosing the right indicators

When you use these indicators, you should choose a subject that is important to you. This may be because you have concerns about your care (e.g. because of a recent significant or critical incident), or because you have recently put effort into a particular aspect of your practice and want to see how well you are doing. Alternatively, you may choose an area that has been suggested as a priority by others, for example, as part of the clinical governance programme of your primary care group/trust, health board or local health group.

Making use of the results

The main purpose of using these indicators is to stimulate discussion. It is unwise to draw definite conclusions about care solely on the basis of using the indicators. There are a number of reasons for this. First, for almost all of the indicators, what we have produced only allows part of the care for that particular condition to be examined. That may be because the panels have not been able to develop indicators (e.g. for aspects of care that are difficult to define), or because there are aspects of care that are not normally recorded in the patient's notes and so are not suitable for record based assessment. So using the indicators should certainly lead you to think, maybe to act, but certainly not to despair!

If you find that the quality of your care appears to be good in terms of the chosen indicators, then you can congratulate yourselves. But you may also wish to think about the following:

▶ Have all the important aspects of care for the chosen condition been considered?

▶ What has been left out?

▶ Are there other aspects of care that cannot be measured, but will benefit from discussion between the doctors and nurses in your practice?

There may be important differences in approach, or things you are uncertain about that don't come out of assessment using the indicators. Nevertheless, using the indicators should help you to talk about the wider aspects of your care.

Deciding on an acceptable standard

In this book, we have not attempted to suggest what standard of care is acceptable. For the majority of conditions, it is unlikely that any practice will score 'full marks' on all the indicators. There may be, for example, good reasons why particular indicators are not applicable to individual patients. On occasions, the standards to be achieved may be set by an external body, as in the case of current target payments for immunisation and cervical cytology. When you are using the indicators in this book to improve care, then it is up to you to decide on what is an acceptable standard for your own population, how much improvement to aim for, and how to balance the effort put into improving quality in one particular condition against other demands in the practice.

What to do if the results look bad

If there appear to be problems in your care, then you need to think about what the indicators are measuring. The most likely problem with any approach that is based on information in medical records is that the information simply isn't there. So, if care seems to fall down in one particular area, you should think first about the following:

- Is the problem that your doctors and nurses are not recording the information in the medical records (computer or Lloyd George)?

- If so, does that matter? The indicators are based on information that our panels of GPs said should definitely be recorded in the patient's notes.

- Is the problem one of computer coding? GP computing systems give scope for substantial variation in the way in which doctors and nurses record care. Do your doctors and nurses all use the same Read codes (or the same as other local practices)? Standardising coding practice makes this type of assessment much easier.

- Does your search strategy need to be changed to take account of the different codes that some doctors or nurses use? Have follow-up consultations been missed, simply because they were not grouped under the original diagnosis on the computer?

- Alternatively, you should consider whether the person who extracted the data may have missed important information. This is particularly important if audits are being carried out using written medical records.

However, the way information is recorded in your notes may be fine, and there may be real problems in the care you provide. This is a judgement that you have to make for yourself. Indicators only 'indicate'. They do not decide. You have to form a value judgement about what the indicators mean. Where care does not reach the standard suggested by the indicators, the literature reviews should be useful in deciding how important that aspect of care is, and what you need to do to change practice.

Using the indicators as evidence for revalidation

Practice teams may use the information derived from the indicators as a guide for their practice development plans but individual general practitioners may also use the indicators to contribute to their personal learning plans as part of their revalidation folder – evidence that they have looked at their own performance. The results do not have to be excellent to contribute to a revalidation folder; what is necessary is for the doctor to show a critical interest in his or her work, and a willingness to learn or institute change. Revalidation folders should contain not only the quantitative results of the assessment but also reflections about what has been learned as a result of the process.

Using the indicators in primary care organisations

The previous section outlined some of the difficulties in using these indicators in individual practices. Larger primary care organisations, such as primary care groups/trusts, local health groups and health boards need to be even more careful in using them to compare different practices.

Why might primary care organisations be interested in using the indicators?

There is likely to be increasing interest in comparisons between practices within primary care organisations. There are two main reasons for this. First, the production and publication of comparative data is being encouraged by the government. For example, the 2000 NHS Plan for England specifically says that information will be produced and published for each practice on its performance against national service frameworks. Second, many primary care organisations are encouraging practices to meet together for education and quality improvement activities, and people have a natural tendency to want to compare themselves with their peers.

Maximising the benefits and reducing the risks of quality indicators

Bearing in mind the pitfalls associated with using indicators outlined above and in chapter 1, how can primary care organisations maximise the likelihood that the indicators will be useful, and minimise the risk of unexpected negative effects?

First, you should only choose issues for investigation where they are important and relevant to the practices involved. Indicators suggested from outside a practice start off at a disadvantage. If they don't even address issues that your practices thinks are important, then the exercise is probably doomed to failure. Practices therefore need to feel a sense of ownership of the agenda. This does not of course mean that primary care organisations should not respond to outside pressures such as nationally set priorities. Indeed, GPs may well find national priorities (e.g. national service frameworks) a useful focus for working together.

Second, primary care organisations need to be aware that all the problems of collecting information on individual practices are compounded when information from different practices is compared. You are likely to find differences in the way information is recorded in different practices. If computer records are used, doctors may use different codes, and it may be difficult to get comparable information from different computer systems. An additional issue arises when different people in different practices have collected the information. Unless you use resources to employ someone to go into practices to collect information, then it is likely that individual staff members will collect information in different ways. Although the indicators in this book have been designed so that they can be collected by trained non-clinicians, the information is probably extracted more reliably by doctors or nurses. The future undoubtedly lies in the electronic extraction of standardised information from computerised records, probably remotely rather than manually or semi-automatically. The MIQUEST search programme is already used to help this process in some areas of the country and the PRIMIS project, based at the University of Nottingham (www.primis.nottingham.ac.uk), is leading developments in this field. However, it is likely to be several years before the technical problems of extracting reliable data remotely are overcome, never mind the ethical issues. In the meantime, practice-based computer searches or manual extraction from medical records will have to suffice.

Case mix and risk adjustment

The circumstances of different practices may also make it difficult for you to make comparisons: a practice that has a high proportion of elderly, sick or socially deprived patients may appear to provide a lower quality of care in comparison with a practice serving a different population. While risk and case mix adjustment is of great importance when comparing relatively rare outcomes, there is considerable debate about the importance of this issue for the kind of indicators described in this book which relate to common technical processes. On one side people argue that case mix adjustment should not be used as an excuse to provide poorer care for certain groups of patients and that the magnitude of the effect of case mix differences on process indicators is not sufficiently large to make adjustment necessary. On the other hand, if definitive judgements are being made on the basis of comparative results, it is only fair to those involved to ensure that there is a level playing field.

The appropriate use of comparative data

Building on the above arguments, the most appropriate response to apparent differences in quality between practices should recognise that:

- Indicators only indicate that the issue is worth looking at in more detail. They do not permit definitive judgements about the quality of care being provided, and they take no account of the important contextual issues that may influence a practice's ability to provide high-quality care. Therefore you should only use them as a basis for further analysis and discussion with practices.

- Comparative information should not be presented in the form of 'league tables'. Some people, particularly those in the media, like the stark comparisons that arise from ranked data. However, these are of dubious scientific value and are unlikely to engage professionals in quality-improvement activities.

- Comparisons are most helpful when made between similar practices – a struggling inner city practice is unlikely to be motivated by comparisons with a leafy suburban practice.

- You may need to spend time and resources to engage practices, the public, health service managers and the media in discussion about the benefits and risks of using quality indicators to compare performance.

Conclusion

Some people may feel that the problems associated with quality indicators are so great that the whole business of collecting and comparing information on quality of care is not worthwhile. This is not our view. While the problems, especially those of data quality and comparability, are great, we believe that the way to improve available information on quality is to start to use it. If judgements start to be made on information that doctors and nurses believe may not be reliable, this can act as a powerful stimulus to change the way in which information is recorded. However, this reinforces the importance of working in areas that are of importance and relevance to the clinicians involved. No one is going to try to improve the way they work for a problem that they regard as irrelevant.

In drawing the indicators together for this book, we hope to have provided some useful tools for those who want to improve the quality of their care. Used carefully, and interpreted with caution, they can form one part of an overall approach to assessing the quality of primary care, demonstrating where good care is being provided and identifying areas where care can be improved.

References

1. Roland MO, Holden J, Campbell S. Quality assessment for general practice: supporting clinical governance in primary care groups. National Primary Care Research and Development Centre, University of Manchester, 1998
2. Roland MO, Baker R. Clinical governance: a guide for primary care teams. National Primary Care Research and Development Centre, University of Manchester, 1999
3. Gask L, Rogers A, Roland M, Morris D. Improving quality in primary care: a practical guide to the National Service Framework for Mental Health. National Primary Care Research and Development Centre, University of Manchester, 2000
4. Cantrill J, Devlin M, Jackson C. Improving quality in primary care: supporting pharmacists working in primary care groups and trusts. National Primary Care Research and Development Centre, University of Manchester, 1999

The text of these handbooks can be downloaded from the website of the National Primary Care Research and Development Centre (www.npcrdc.man.ac.uk).